THE ESSENTIAL
MARTIN BLACK

VOLUME NO. 1

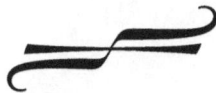

HORSEBACK

ISBN 978-0-9600259-2-3

Table of Contents

Introduction

Quite often when visiting with horse people I hear comments like, "Yeah but you don't understand; these are Thoroughbred horses," or, "But this is a Dressage horse," or "Yeah, but mate, this is a Campdrafter." The fact is, all horses are limited by their bio-mechanics, neurological systems, and gravitational forces. Which means they only move in certain ways, they only react in certain ways, and they only balance in certain ways, regardless of breed or discipline.

This doesn't mean that all horses are the same. What it does mean is that there are consistencies in horses. And there are consistent misunderstandings people have with them. They are prey animals; we are predators by nature. They understand this which makes them easy to intimidate. In the proper dosage, this can be very useful to us getting them to yield to the slightest pressure, physical or mental.

They operate from self-preservation much more than we do. They try to get away from pressure, which is their flight mode. If they cannot get away, they go against pressure which is a fight mode. When we do not engage their self preservation, they seek comfort.

When we put them through this process, they learn how to avoid the discomfort and find comfort. This is the major motivator for them to learn the patterns that we find beneficial—to give to pressure.

There are certain things that most all horses are going to be required to do when we ride them: move forward, move left, move right, stop, and possibly back up. There may be certain levels of refinement to move in particularly ways, but it starts with these basics. And quite often the problem with the higher level horses is that they don't have the basics down very well.

There are certain things we need from a horse to be safe and useful from the ground also. They are big, they are strong, and they are quick. This can make them very dangerous to us. They don't mean to be, and they don't want to be dangerous, but it happens. It happens because of the lack of understanding on our part for their need of self-preservation.

Horses have no ego, they have no greed, and they have no prejudice. This makes their decision making quite different than ours. The better we understand this the better we can see things from their perspective and understand why they do what they do.

These short articles are examples of this philosophy. Depending on where you are in your understanding of horsemanship you can be exposed to new ideas at different times and they will have a different meaning. An experience you have now will not have the same learning opportunity that it would have had previously or in the future. You will observe a situation or read material at different times and you can get different things from it.

Good luck and I hope you find something here that will benefit you.

ACKNOWLEDGMENTS

I would like to thank all the people smarter than me that helped me to put this material together. Through the years that I have written these articles, there has been different people editing them trying to decipher my bad grammar and bad spelling. Emily Kitching is one of these people and she is also the one that has spurred me more than anyone to write these. And also Kim Stone for a lot of very nice photography and support through the years. I would much rather be on a horse with a rope in my hand than at a desk with pen or IPad.

Thank you.
Martin Black

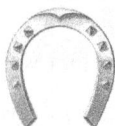

What Do You Mean by Soft Feel?

*W*hat are people talking about when they mention "a soft feel"?

What I believe a soft feel is referring to is when the rider draws on the reins and the horse responds with out any resistance through the body down to the feet. At the same time the horse should respond likewise to the riders' legs, seat and body rhythm.

What I see in a big percent of riders is that the horse may be responsive to the bit. When the reins tighten, the horse gives in the poll and the nose comes back vertically. Some will have horizontal flexion when the feet are stopped.

What I like to see is the "soft feel" or light contact carry through not only in the walk and trot, stopping backing and making circles, but at any speed and any maneuver. The same soft feel we have with the reins, we should have with our legs. If we develop enough feel with our hands and legs and our horse is familiar with the job we are asking, we should be able to use a lot of body language or rhythm and our horse can follow us just like we are leading a dance and they are following. We shouldn't need a lot of obvious communication if our dancing partner is assertive and willing. But at the same time, we develop a feel or rhythm to stay together, one leading, one following.

We don't need to be desensitizing a horse to the point that we have to use pain or fear to get a response. This can get in the way of maintaining a soft feel. The horse needs to be safe but we shouldn't need to make him unresponsive. The more experience we have, the more we can anticipate what the horse's response or next move will be and the more we can enhance or inhibit his thoughts and actions in the direction we want. It is a lot easier to maintain the soft feel with a horse if we have life in his feet. It is hard to direct a horse that isn't moving, or isn't moving willingly.

When a horse is moving you can adjust the comfort areas to help him learn to follow you. He will seek comfort. It takes relief for pressure to be effective and pressure for relief to be effective. One of the arts of horsemanship is to find and refine a balance between pressure and relief. You don't need to use pain or fear to get a response.

Most horses are going to start out being uncomfortable with a rider on their back that is not in rhythm with their movement. If the rider is tight or not in sync with the horse, the horse will not be as content as if the rider's movement offers no resistance to the horse.

If we start out with a horse that is tight, whether it is a green horse that is unsure of his well-being or an experienced horse that is sure of his well-being, we should first get the horse confident that he can relax and we can have one rhythm like dancers. You need to get with his rhythm first, then start altering his movement to get him with your movement.

This may mean if the horse is too confused and can't follow what you are expecting of him, you need to get with him— we need to learn to go with the horse until the horse can learn to go with the person. Drop back to a level that he can be more comfortable with. The horse is always willing if he is confident he can maintain comfort, which is the major motivator for a horse. Fear causes them to react out of self-preservation; this is a reaction not a thought process. Pain causes them to resist or protect themselves and if they cannot find protection they accept and tolerate the pain. Although pain can get a thoughtful response, it usually isn't a willing response.

The more sensitive we are (every time we touch the horse), the more the horse can be sensitive to us in a positive way and this is when we can develop the soft feel. We have to develop a feel with our horse before we can develop a soft feel.

The horse will have this soft feel if we don't cause resistance. The horse will not resist comfort, this is the major motivator in a horses' life. What he looks forward to in life is comfort. If we can learn how to offer him comfort and show him how to avoid discomfort, he will follow a soft feel with us.

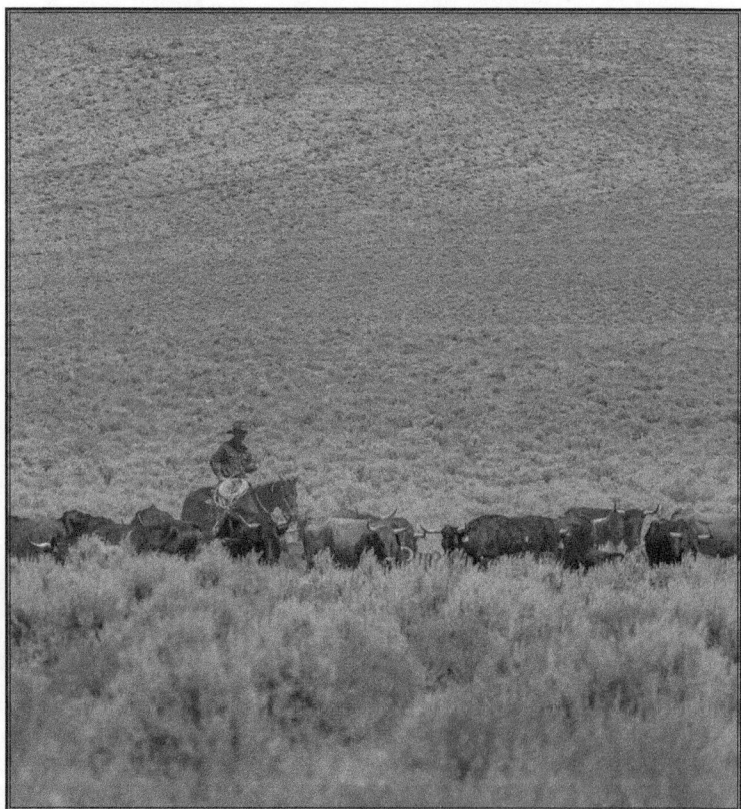

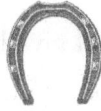

OPEN THE GATE

eing able to open a gate from your horse can be very useful and perhaps necessary for some who have trouble getting off and on their horse.

For those riders that may have trouble, breaking the exercise down into separate components may help. By doing so, you may identify one small part of the process that is missing. First, the horse must have some appreciation for standing, or what I like to call "parking." To me this is important for a lot of other reasons. The horse should stand or park until he is asked otherwise. To establish this, position the horse next to the gate where you can reach the latch and release any pressure you are applying with your hands or legs to hold him there. If the horse starts to walk off, let him take a few steps, then sidepass or back him around a few seconds and come back to the same position you had him parked originally. If the horse walks off again, repeat the process and maybe work him around just a little longer before putting him back into position.

The idea is to relax and give him relief at the gate and make work for him out of trying to go anywhere else. In the process the horse can get handier at moving his feet in different directions, and then appreciate the relief you are offering when he stands or parks next to the gate. In the end he should only move off when you ask him to, not when he decides to.

Once park is established, some horses may have trouble staying balanced and not moving their feet when the rider's weight transfers from center to the side. To establish this, just lean to one side, then the other, coming back to center, if you can, just before the horse moves his feet. Transferring a small amount of weight will teach the horse to brace against it, and then going back and forth will give him time to prepare for more each time with some relief while passing center each time.

This brace we built to lean is the same brace that helps a horse to stand while mounting and dismounting. When the horse can brace while you lean without leaving, he is ready for the next step.

The next step would be to get the horse to accept the movement and noise of the gate. It's helpful to have a gate that is balanced and only moves when you move it and doesn't fall to the same spot. While the horse is parked, lean over and just move the gate back and forth a few inches. If the horse is going to move, try to stop moving the gate before he moves and give him time to evaluate and accept the gate moving. Then keep increasing the movement and noise until he accepts it at any level. Then move the gate and step one step toward it and stop. Give him some time to evaluate what happened and do it again.

If at all possible, position your horse from the start so the gate swings away from him and he goes through the gate headfirst or going forward. Do Not pull the gate into a green horse and bump his feet or let him think the gate is chasing him. If and when he gets away, you just taught him to outrun this uncertain object. And Do Not try backing the horse through the gate. If the horse is uncertain of the situation, and then you ask him to move and he can't see where he is going, you will cause more uncertainty and resistance. Step the horse sideways and forward into the gate so he can see where he is going and where the post and gate is.

The key is to make parking a safe place. Then if the horse becomes uncertain, he can stop and find relief, then start again. This idea can be applied in several areas. Stop when you get lost, think about it, and then start again.

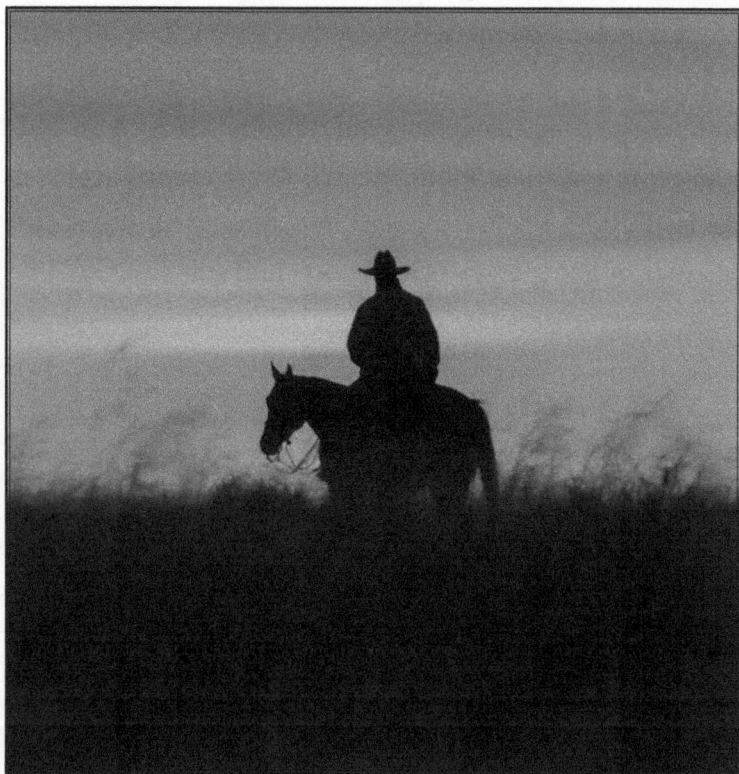

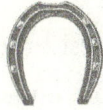

Devoloping the Stop

Getting a horse to stop isn't only necessary in most riding disciplines but is also a safety precaution at some point for most all riders if things ever get out of control. If a horse doesn't understand to stop, it can be difficult to check his speed to prevent a hazardous situation.

There are various ways to develop a stop and various ways for a horse to stop for various reasons. I am not going to get into the finer points of a big sliding stop on the hindquarters or what I call a cowhorse stop, which the horse uses all four quarters to stop. We need to develop the idea, the basic concept first, and from that we can refine a high-performance stop.

This simple exercise can help with an older horse that isn't putting out much effort or a young inexperienced horse that just doesn't know. One thing the rider needs to understand is how we affect the horse's balance and natural way of moving and operating when we pull hard enough that the horse engages muscles to resist the pull. The other response is when the horse is supple enough to overflex or get too much bend that he has to transfer the weight on the front and the hindquarters to compensate for his head and neck in an unnatural position.

With a light enough pull on the reins, and keeping our weight close to the center of gravity into and through the stop, the horse can perform with the least distraction from us and find out how to balance himself to stop.

The idea of this exercise is to find a speed (probably a trot or a slow lope) that will cause the horse to work a little, but not get confused. Once he works for a while, and realizes the pressure is consistent and the relief is also consistent, he will avoid the pressure area and want to stay in the relief area you are offering. The concept to remember is: It takes relief for pressure to be effective, and pressure for relief to be effective. The balance of these two will develop a confident, compliant, and motivated horse. When he experiences too much relief, he will be lazy, resentful, or bored. When he experiences too much pressure he can become nervous, mad, frustrated, confused, or over anticipate the maneuver. Using good judgment in this area will determine your success or failure.

To set this exercise up, find an area with good footing where you can make a circle that you will complete approximately every ten seconds or so. This timing allows the horse enough time to relax between maneuvers without losing his train of thought.

As you come in a circle to the left, pick a spot to stop and roll back to the right, then you will make a right circle and come to the exact same spot, stop and roll back to the left and make another left circle and continue with this. Each circle will be on top of the last, and each stop will be in the same spot. As you ask your horse to stop, your body rhythm will stop; then just take the slack out of the reins. If you feel better saying whoa, that's fine, but he will read your body rhythm also.

Choose a speed that with a light pull on the reins would bring your horse to a walk in around four steps. Just one or two steps before the horse slows to a walk, pull one rein just hard enough to elevate the head but not panic the horse. If the horse panics, he will respond without thinking, but if he doesn't elevate the head he is not acknowledging the discomfort, and this is what is going to motivate him to look for a more comfortable deal. When you affect the horse properly, this should only take a few times to make a slight change, and the horse should start putting more effort into the stop. When you see the change, don't roll back, but just stop and wait for the horse to relax. Put your hands on his neck and let your reins long to let your horse know you quit for that session and try again later.

Remember, to look for the effort to reward, and do not prepare to pull the reins. He may take a deep breath or lick his lips. He is fully realizing the relief at this point and this is going to motivate him to put effort in the stop and be relaxed and confident. After two or three slight improvements, quit for the day, and don't get hung up on looking for a certain level of performance.

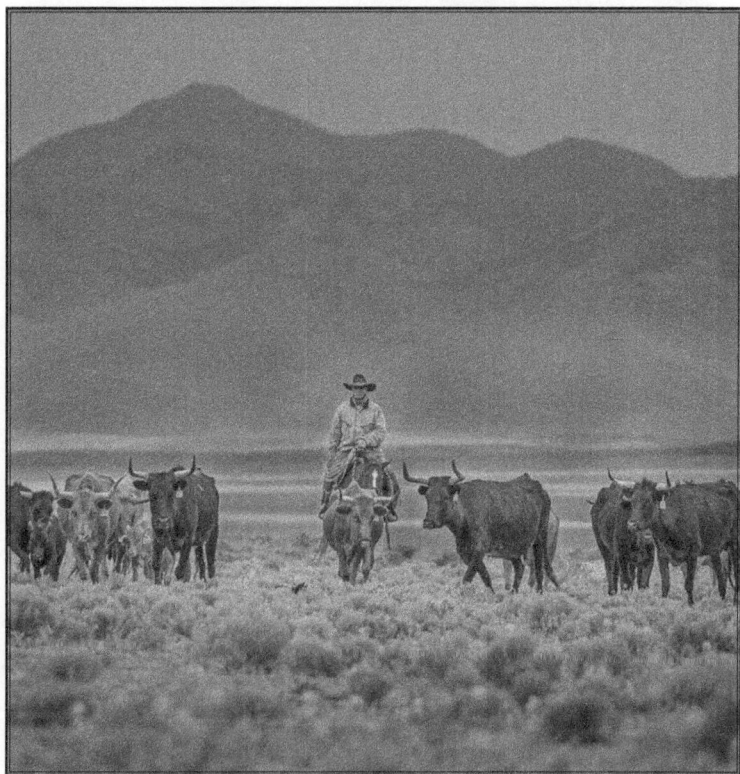

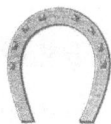

DOUBLING AND ITS IMPORTANCE

Doubling isn't a maneuver you would see in a reining pattern, dressage class, cow horse event, or any other advanced performance competitions. But if it is the first maneuver a horse learns and maintains properly, it can help prevent a lot of mishaps and undesirable patterns.

The horse needs to learn to perform this maneuver properly and completely; bits and pieces now and then will only give the horse and rider a false sense of security. Different people may have a different interpretation or understanding of doubling; I will define mine and the importance of it.

Starting with the tip of the horse's nose, regardless of whether the colt was started in a snaffle, hackamore, or halter, as the slack is drawn out of the rein, the horse should tip his nose toward the rein with a slight bend in the poll. One of the most important things to look for is if the horse is supple in the poll. If the horse is not supple in the poll, he will not be supple in the loin and he will be braced mentally. All three work together, simultaneously, and no training device can get this until the horse is ready to give it. Most horses will give this with very little challenge if we haven't given them a reason to be defensive. A horse can bend his neck until their nose touches the saddle but if the poll is straight the loin will be also, Mentally he is defensive, his guard is up so he is ready to push forward with the hindquarters. The poll is straight so he can see a flight path.

The shoulder can be falling to the outside or to the inside; in either case this can be a dangerous position to be in. The horse will be pushing forward with the hind feet extending back more than a normal stride, which puts more weight on the front feet. The horse is not balanced in any sense of the word, and if the horse were to stumble in front, it's difficult to make a recovery because the other three feet are behind the center of gravity. Again loin, poll, and mind all working simultaneously is like having three different meters. If you can read one, the other two will read the same. In most of the defensive maneuvers a horse uses against us, running, bucking, rearing, etc., the hindquarters are engaged, and locked, and the loin is straight.

When the horse is broke in the poll, and in the loin, and if the nose is pointed to some degree to the left, the hind feet will be stepping to the right. When the horse can do this consistently and with some confidence, the inside hind feet will be reaching up under toward the girth, and the inside front would be stepping shortest or pivoting while the other three feet maintain a forward motion. Regardless of how this is achieved, to me there is little room to compromise. This is the one thing that will help ensure you don't lose control and most importantly, maintain safety for the rider and horse before leaving the round pen.

Some horses while moving in a straight line at a slow pace may stop the front feet or even step them back when the hind feet step out. This will not benefit the doubling because the horse may have trouble going from a forward motion with speed and shift his weight back if he is too scared to stop in front so the hind feet can step out.

If the horse knows how to step the hind feet out while at any speed, the horse can be doubled; and because the feet are reaching forward, they can maintain their balance. The slower the horse is going, the farther he can reach out, but at any speed he can disengage or quit pushing with the hind-quarters and shift them to the outside of the line of travel. When done properly, the doubling maneuver can prevent a horse from bucking or running out of control and, with a slightly different presentation, can help prepare the horse for a rollback or a sliding stop later on.

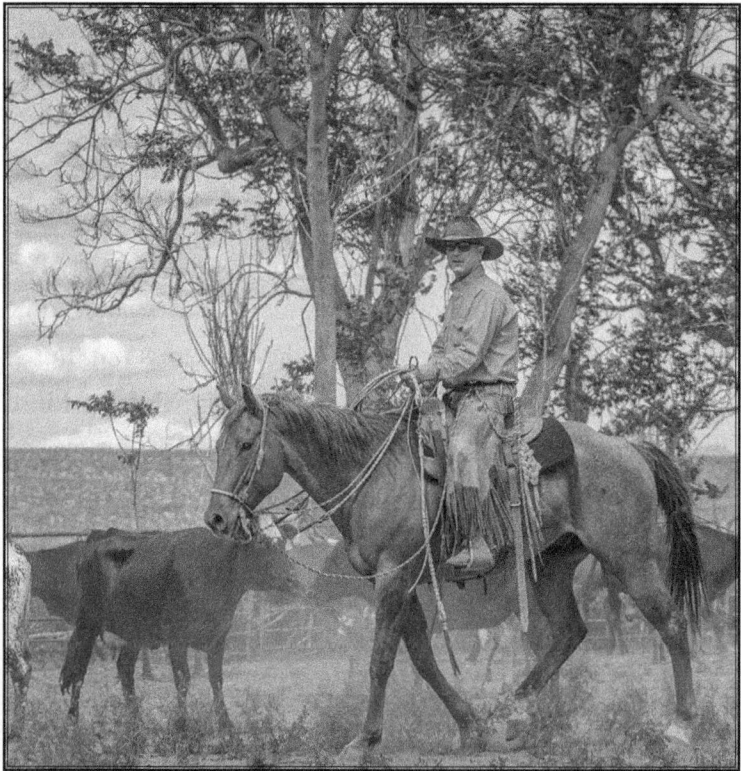

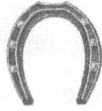

GET BACK

The majority of a horse's movement is in a forward motion. If something is causing a loose horse to back up, he will usually shift his weight back, then turn and move away in a forward motion. The horse's inherent instinct is to run away from danger, and he can easily see behind him at a distance, so he will not hesitate to run if threatened.

A horse may back straight and not turn if he is more curious than threatened, but it would be unusual for the horse to get much experience without a person handling him to keep him straight. With this in mind, when we want to get our horse to back straight for an extended length, it will take some understanding on the part of the person to acknowledge that this is one thing the horse has little experience doing.

If we watch different horses and analyze what is taking place, some look like the rider is trying to push a chain; parts are going every direction. The head may go up in the air, or tuck under toward the chest; the shoulders may go to the left or right; and the hips may go to one side or the other also, but not straight back. Other horses can back and look like the chain is being pulled with every link moving exactly on the same line. In this case the horse's spine will be exactly straight from the tip of the tail to the poll, and the poll may not have any vertical flexion. Why? Because the horse has engaged the hindquarters to pull "the chain" before the rider puts too much pressure on the head trying to push "the chain."

How do we get this? First, the rider needs to understand what makes the difference and what it feels like. It may be easier to learn what it feels like if another person is visually helping. It is as simple as knowing if the hind feet are moving before the front or if the front feet are moving before the hind. In other words, the front starts to push the hind, "pushing a chain," or the hind pulls the front, "pulling a chain." If the hind foot leaves the ground before the opposite front, the hind will be pulling, or if the hind and front leave simultaneously at least the hind is not causing resistance. The resistance is what you feel in the pushing scenario that would be when the front foot moves before the opposite hind foot.

If the horse is light and supple with the hindquarters moving from side to side, it will be easier to move him back. Start by putting just enough pressure on the reins that the horse acknowledges you. This means the slightest movement of the head, up, down, looking back to one side, anything. Then put one leg on his side to move the hindquarters over; use one rein to reinforce only if necessary. As soon as the hind foot steps over one step, move the hindquarters back over the other way one step. All we are trying to do is step the hindquarters left and right one step from side to side. If the horse moves forward, be firm on the reins until he is back in his original tracks; then resume the light pressure. If the reins are swinging real free, without stopping, and the horse hasn't stepped back, just put a little more pressure on the reins to see if he will shift his weight back. When he does take a step, just sit still for at least as long as the horse worked leading up to taking a step back so he can realize how he got out of the situation. Two or three minutes wouldn't be too long. This may be a good time to get on the cell phone.

One thing that will make a difference is if the rider will take all the weight out of the seat and stand with their weight more on the stirrups or thighs. When the feet are moving, the horse will raise the loin easier and thus make it easier to position and use the hindquarters. With some practice, and not violating the horse's confidence, you can get older horses backing better, or get a colt to come back the first step. It's just a matter of getting the hind feet started first.

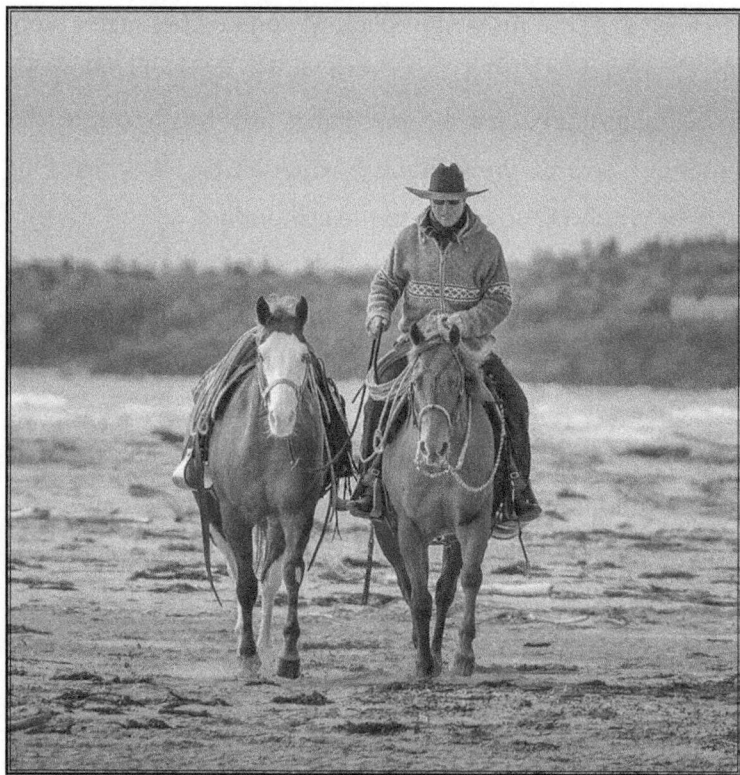

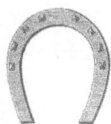

Straighten
That Horse Out

How straight can you ride your horse? If you think your horse can ride in a straight line, pick an object like a fence post 50 or 100 yards in front of you and another object farther away, maybe a power pole or a spot on a ridge. These two fixed objects can be your sights. See if you can ride for 50 or 100 yards with your horse going straight without you needing to help. If it feels like your paddling upstream with one oar, you can work on this to see if you can get it feeling like your paddling downstream with two oars.

First of all, a person needs to stay focused. You can't drive a car straight looking at the hood ornament. You need to be looking out ahead of you a hundred yards or more to send the car straight. As the road pulls you one way, you can make a slight correction earlier the farther you are looking ahead. When you ride your horse in this manner, you are giving your horse a more precise objective. If you can be clear on where you want to go, and aware of how your horse is interpreting this objective, your horse will likely put his ears forward and be looking for what you are looking at. Then you will be looking directly between your horse's ears to your two targets with all three lined up.

This may not come quick or easy, but the more consistent and persistent you are, the better you can develop this and the more enjoyable your horse will go somewhere for you and the easier some performance maneuvers will be to work on also. To get a high-performance straight sliding stop, your horse needs to be running dead straight. To send a rope horse to a cow, he needs to run straight, and you need to be able to communicate this desire to your horse to be right when you get where you are going.

You can find many ways to get this accomplished, and I will just try to give you some thoughts that might help. Think of yourself riding your horse down the bottom of a ditch, the sides slope up gradually and get steeper until they are very difficult to negotiate. When your horse is traveling in the bottom of this ditch, that should be the least resistance. As you vary off your line and the bottom, it becomes more difficult as the slope increases. But as you come down the slope toward the center, it immediately becomes easier. If you pass the center and start out the other side, you run into more resistance until you start back down toward the center.

Don't pressure your horse to the line, only while he is going away from the line. If he can interpret that he is running into his own pressure, it will make sense to him. But if he feels pressure going away and pressure coming back he just learns to tolerate it as nonsense. When your horse can feel your support to stay in the middle with you, follow the path of least resistance, reinforced by the knowledge of running into his own pressure, the choice is easy for him. You can use your reins, your outside leg to push him over, your inside leg to bend him back. It doesn't matter what or how he gets into trouble. The important thing is he interprets the trouble with leaving the line and the relief with hunting to stay on the line.

Once you develop this with your horse, you will be able to send him straight down the arena, straight to the far ridge, or keep your focus to one side slightly, and he can make a round circle. After you are able to turn him loose to go where you want and he only meets resistance when he varies right or left, he will follow your arc like he followed your straight line.

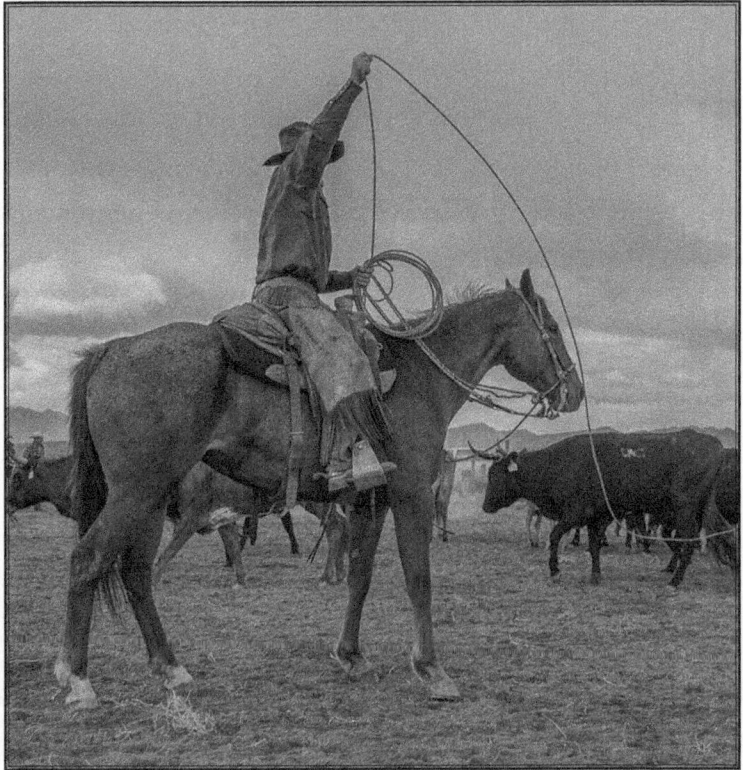

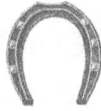

Prepare For the Hackamore and Bridle

The Spanish-type hackamore and bridle are both traditionally designed to operate from feel not force. When they become a forceful tool, the outcome will be reversed from the original intent.

Both the hackamore and bridle put pressure on the outside, the jaw and the neck, which if yielding to pressure, the horse will tip the nose to the outside. When he has learned to follow a feel, the nose will tip in the direction of travel while turning and the horse will stay balanced. When these tools are used forcefully as leverage devices, the leverage of both the hackamore and a neck rein on a bridle will tip the nose to the outside while pulling the neck to the inside. Two things that tell the tale if the horse has been brought along with understanding is first, the poll will be supple, and second, the jaw will be relaxed, not clenched.

In order for a horse to accept the bridle, he cannot be intimidated by it. When a horse is started properly and brought along through the hackamore and two-rein, a lot of time is spent for the horse to learn through experience and not fear. Bits that inflict pain such as tongue relief and that pressure the more sensitive bars of a horse's mouth cause the horse to raise his head initially, especially with a quick movement from the reins.

A straight bar lying across the horse's tongue, like the traditional Spanish bits, allows the horse to hold the bit off the bars by flexing the tongue and holding the bit. A roller or cricket encourages the horse to work his tongue by giving him something to play with. He learns to enjoy the sound of a loud cricket, and when we pick the reins up, he can pick up the bit and roll the cricket which helps him to keep his mouth moist and his jaw relaxed.

Young horses that have not had their mouths violated by harsh bits or harsh hands will learn to enjoy and play with the bit. The horse that dreads the movement of quick or heavy hands or more severe bits will not likely, if ever, play with and enjoy the bit.

When we push a horse beyond his confidence level, especially when training him in the hackamore or bridle, to the point of fear and confusion, we must be very careful and back out of that area to minimize the damages. When the horse loses his confidence and we punish him and cause panic or resentment, we may create a situation that could take a multitude of good experiences to offset the one bad experience, and he may never trust that it won't happen again.

We cannot force a horse to relax. When his self-preservation is engaged they are tense, tight, flighty, and maybe even fighting. He needs to be confident that his safety is not being jeopardized, not just in his work, but free from pain being inflicted on him from quick or heavy hands. Pain and especially quick, unexpected pain or a surprise makes it difficult for the horse to relax.

A very simple test is to take one rein to bring the head laterally. The one eye should look up the rein, while the face remains somewhat vertical, not looking away, and the head should not start toward a horizontal position. When you ask for vertical flexion, he should break in the poll without elevating the head first.

The horse can bend his neck laterally and vertically without bending his poll.

Bending the horse's neck does not mean he is supple in the poll. Flexing should be a test, not an exercise. When the horse has the proper preparation and understanding, there is no reason for his poll not to be supple.

In the training of a hackamore and bridle horse, a supple poll is the trademark of a horse that has learned to accept and operate with these traditional tools the way they were intended.

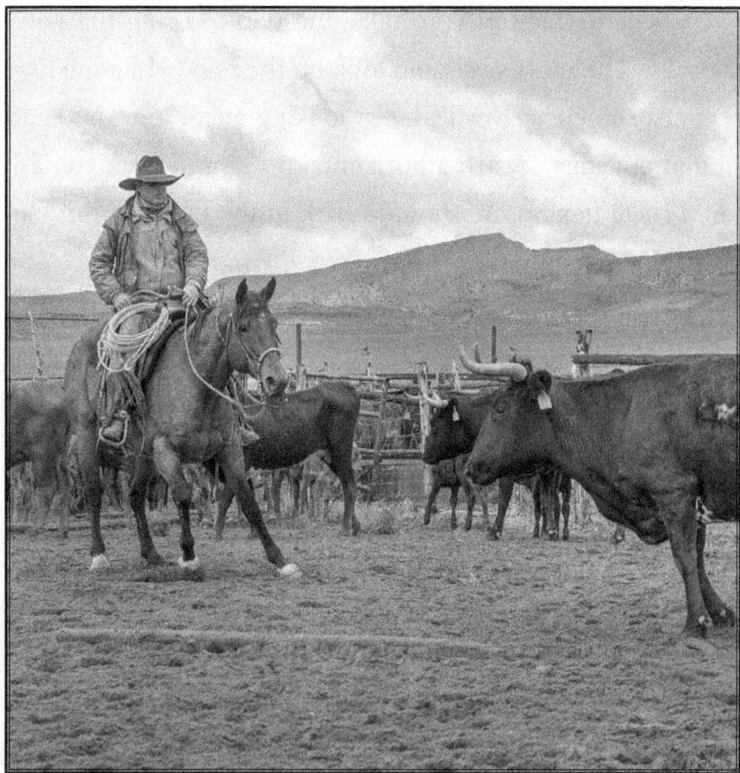

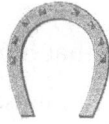

LET THE COW WORK
YOUR HORSE

*O*f all the techniques, methods and gimmicks to get our horses to do what we want, one of my favorites has always been a cow. By making position comfortable for the horse, whether it be offense or defense, we can encourage him to move at different speeds and direction with a purpose.

The laws of nature are relatively simple and consistent that animals live by, although they are different for predators than for prey animals. That's where the problem for us humans comes in. We think as predators, but we need to try to reason with the horse, thinking as a prey animal. We need to understand how prey animals think, and reason with them accordingly.

Some of the basic laws that horses naturally live by are:

1. Horses are herd animals; they go to their mother or the herd for security.

2. They have a flight or comfort zone. This is the area around them, that, when penetrated, engages their self-preservation.

3. They respond to pressure and relief, mentally, emotionally and physically.

4. As prey animals, they are always cautious of aggressive actions by others.

5. Their first defense is flight, if they don't feel that option is available, they fight.

By understanding and applying these principles, our communication can be much easier for our horses and us. Horses are instinctively drawn to the herd. Their earliest experiences naturally are to move to and with the herd when they experience any suspicion of danger. If we can apply this into our working with horses, the message is much clearer and we can capitalize on knowledge and experience the horse already has.

For example, to get a green horse to move out, we need a cow that will move away as the horse approaches. Then we can relax any pressure we are applying when the horse looks or moves toward the cow. When the horse's attention is not on the cow, or he is committed to moving away from the cow, apply pressure to the horse. The horse will feel relief toward the cow, and discomfort away from the cow. This will motivate the horse to go to the cow for comfort as he has experienced in the past with his mother or the herd for comfort and security. When he makes this connection, it is like he instantly gained a lot of training, but in reality, we have just shown him he can use some of what he already has learned to make his life easier. With the cow leading us, we can get some direction and speed variance.

Another example is getting a green horse to turn on the hindquarters. We need to tap the horse's knowledge on flight zones. The horse will have one and the cow will have one, since both of them are prey animals. Flight Zone is the area around an animal that when something approaches too close, they feel the need to move to maintain a safe distance.

If the cow is drawn toward the horse by wanting to return to the other cattle, or because the cow is against a fence, we will be able to engage the cow's flight zone.

A fence corner or wings at about 30 degrees off parallel of each other is useful. The more the horse pushes the cow into the corner or narrow end of the pen, the more the fences pressure the cows' flight zone. The closer the horse is, the more the horse pressures its flight zone. The cow is not going through the fence, so it tries to come past the horse. The only way to maintain position on the cow is to get away from it or get out of the flight zone. By taking the pressure away, the cow will slow down or stop, allowing the horse to slow down or stop. The horse can learn from this application that by pressuring the cow into the corner, he creates work for himself. When the horse gets out of the cow's flight zone, and the cow stops, we need to let the horse stop, relax, and air up if needed. This pause will motivate the horse to look this position up next time things speed up. When we step in to turn the cow, if the horse turns with forward motion, we get deeper into the cow's flight zone and the cow will speed up. This causes more work or pressure for the horse because the horse now has to speed up. We can help the horse learn that he can slow the cow down by staying out of the cow's flight zone, or moving away from the cow.

We can put pressure on the horse with our legs and reins when the cow is close. The horse will interpret this like it is coming from the cow and it will encourage him to keep the cow out of his flight zone, then we offer relief when the cow is out of the horse's flight zone. Since we are applying the pressure, based on our position with the cow, we determine where the horse's flight zone is.

When this starts working, we can ride toward the cow until it moves then let the horse get out of the cow's flight zone. With this, we can develop a stop and a back because the horse does not want to approach the cow's flight zone and the horse wants to keep the cow out of his flight zone.

We can set up a turn when the cow is moving into the horse. This means we are pressuring the flight zone of the cow and the horse. As the cow turns into the horse, the horse will want to get back away from the cow's flight zone and protect his own flight zone. The horse will then pull back, making a turn over the hindquarters.

The other main component that animals operate from is a balance point. This is the point that we influence the cow to change directions or stop. When the cow's flight zone is engaged, and its route is blocked and the animal still chooses to travel or escape, it will choose another route. When the flight zone is not engaged or the animal's safety is not threatened, we can block the cow's balance point and we can stop the cow.

Again, the horse will already know about balance point if he has had the opportunity to play or fight with other horses in the past. Whether he is aggressive or submissive to another horse, the position from the left or the right of the balance point will determine the direction. The depth of the flight zone will determine the speed. He can be on offense or defense, delivering or receiving, and they will have experienced these components.

When we understand this experience and knowledge the horse already possesses before we influence him, and let him put this to our benefit, we can get ahead of the game quick.

The cow basically becomes an object that the horse is cautious to crowd. By approaching the cow, we can step up stops, turns, and backing, using the flight zone to pressure the horse and offering relief at the balance point of the cow.

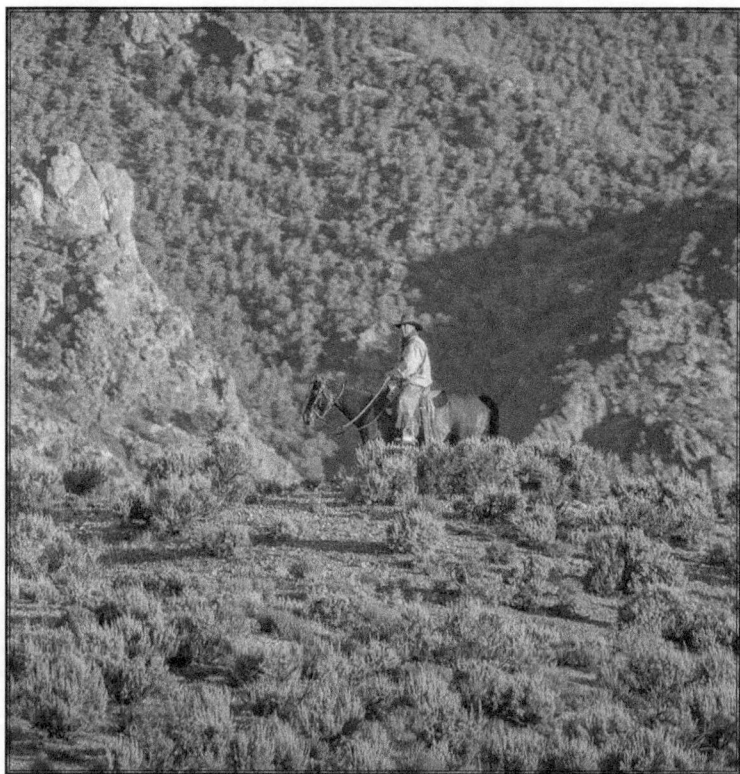

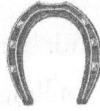

Stop Holding On

*I*n the making of a Hackamore or Bridle Horse, the quality of the finished product will depend greatly on the timing and feel offered by the hands on the reins. We can use different bits, hackamores or other devices tied at different angles to develop a head set or certain responses, but the maintenance is going to come down to how well we can present and maintain a feel with our hands.

If it was easy, anybody could do it. But, it isn't, and that is why we have to work to figure it out. What we can learn from other horseman may work at certain times, however every situation may be different. We need to develop our judgment, so we are able to compensate under any circumstance.

One thing that makes a lot of situations difficult for the horse is when the person holds steady pressure on the reins for a complete maneuver. We can only pull or send a signal and expect the horse to respond as the foot or feet are on the ground or leaving the ground. The horse can not redirect a foot that is falling. If we are pulling as the horses' foot is coming down, he can only wear the pull until the foot is on the ground again and then reposition for a change. This is the point which the horse can easily learn to push on our hands. It is important that we slack or relax the pressure on the reins when the horse can comply and get in time with the feet to apply pressure when the horse can comply. A big percent of the problems people have when handling their horses is a result of their feel and timing not being compatible to the horse. This causes problems with head position and/or being hard mouthed.

An insecure horse may require a light, steady contact to support the idea to complete a maneuver, but too much force from the reins can be counter productive.

The more experience the horse has, the better the horse should understand his job. The more the horse understands his job, the less we should need to do. We need to be patient and understanding with the horse that does not have confidence. At the same time we need to be careful, yet effective, with the horse that doesn't have the motivation or desire. Only experience will teach us to recognize the difference.

We can't expect the horse to give us our desired response if we can't communicate what it is. They haven't learned to communicate our way in the last thousand years, but there is record of people being successful in communicating with the horse in a way they understand. We need to be open to what may work for them—not arrogant and forceful of what we want to make happen. There is a point at which the pressure we may apply with the reins passes from being a respected signal to being a resented signal. No one knows where this point is except on a case by case or step by step basis.

When asking our horse to do anything, there are different levels of response that we should look for. Be aware of the processes that take place before the full force of the pull is delivered, and the horse gives us a full response.

The first level will be acknowledgement: when the horse realizes there may be a signal coming and may evaluate or prepare to respond. This may be a time that could pay off for us if we wait and feel for a change in the horse, instead of dragging or pushing him through the maneuver. Wait and see if he can find it and follow through on his own. If he can, it may feel good enough to him that the experience could promote him to look forward to doing it again when you give a light signal.

The next level is when the horse prepares to respond. He shifts his weight, repositions his body, or in some way alters what he was doing in a positive or desirable way. This is definitely when we want to do as little as possible. Get the job done, but make it as good of an experience as possible for the horse to encourage him to take the same avenue next time we present the situation again.

If we do not recognize and encourage our horses' small efforts, we find ourselves at the next level: when the horse feels he cannot find a comfortable solution to escape the pressure he is experiencing. The horse can push against our hands, or alter his head position, which can alter his balance and make it difficult for him to be collected and easy for him to drop his shoulders. When he is distracted enough to get off balance, he is probably distracted enough to forget about working a cow or any other project we were trying to direct his attention toward.

At this point, based on his past experience and, to some extent his genetic makeup, he responds with confusion, fear, frustration, anger, resentment or other emotional responses—all of which could need to be responded to by us individually. What causes confusion or fear in one horse may cause frustration or resentment in another. This is why it is important to diagnose the specific problem properly before prescribing a cure, and to be sure you are treating the cause and not the symptom.

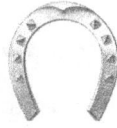

WHERE ARE THOSE FEET GOING?

If we don't have jobs for our horse we need to create some. A horse seems to do better in his learning if he can have a purpose. The better our judgment is on how much to expect of him the more productive our time can be while he is learning.

Whether we are doing a real job or we create a job, we need to have some level of control so that we can position our horse to open a gate, cross a creek, work a cow, etc. Sometimes the success of the job may depend on a correct step, or even a half step in the correct direction.

The speed of the movement can be important. Whether the hind quarters, the front quarters or both of them at the same time can be moved laterally in the same direction or in opposite directions may determine the success of the job we need to get done. We need to be able to move each end

39

or both ends any direction. A good exercise to develop some communication between us and the horse is to pick a pivot foot and move the other three feet around it, without moving the pivot foot. Without some practice, this can even be a challenge for a broke horse.

Pick the right front foot and keep weight on it, so it does not leave the ground. Then with the other three feet moving forward and over, turn the horse around 360 degrees. Easy enough? Then with the other three feet stepping backwards, turn 360 degrees.

The ultimate goal is to be able to rotate the horse forward or backward and full circle while pivoting on each of the four feet. In order to do this, we have to be able to not only feel what feet are moving what direction, but feel the weight shifting before the feet move. If we wait to see what foot moves, it may be too late to stop or redirect the other feet the direction we need to go.

If we have trouble with this, a couple of things can help. One is to have someone be your eyes for you. If you are trying to look at what the feet are doing, you won't be focusing on feeling what the feet are doing the way you need to be. Try to feel what the feet are preparing to do and have someone call out what is actually happening.

Feel the withers tip right, left, forward or backwards. Feel the hip shift right, left, forward or backwards. The horse will shift his weight in order to prepare to move each foot. If the weight isn't positioning correctly, the feet are not going to follow through correctly.

We need to develop enough feel to know what is shaping

up with the horse. The horse needs to develop enough feel with our hands, legs and weight in order to understand what we are trying to shape up.

The other thing is to only move one or two steps and evaluate what happened. Whether you are alone or have some one calling steps for you, focus on what you feel, then add the visual to the equation.

Another thing this can do is to focus on the first step being the step we need. If we need to step the hind feet forward and to the right, and the front takes two or three steps before the hind can move for us, this may wreck what we were trying to position for.

Whether your horse did what you were asking or not, evaluate how he started out and how he interpreted what you were asking. If you are getting too much forward motion when he feels your leg, you may need to shift his weight back to ensure contact and to convey the message that you are ready to block forward movement, so the leg can be interpreted for lateral movement.

If the front end moves laterally before the hind end, shift the weight off the front end one direction first with the reins. Then try to move the hind end the opposite direction with your leg.

Again, if the movement doesn't start right, stop, evaluate what you did, how the horse responded to it, and then try again. Don't panic and get in a hurry. If you are going the wrong direction and you speed up, you just get to the wrong place quicker.

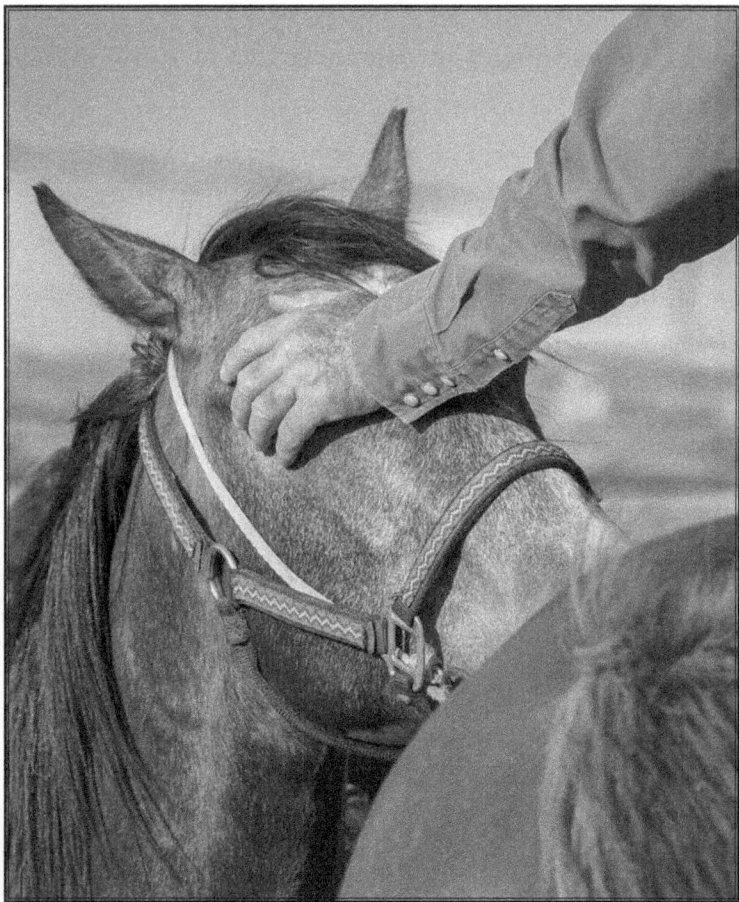

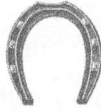

FLIGHT OR FIGHT? YIELD OR RESIST?

*W*e have all heard it said that *"A horse's first means of defense is flight, and his second means of defense is to fight."*

Then we hear: "It's natural for a horse to go against pressure." Or, "Giving to pressure is against a horse's nature, he has to be taught to yield to pressure."

Which way is it? These statements sound like opposites to me. Wouldn't a horse be yielding by running away, and fighting when he goes against pressure? When a horse is free from any confinement, and we put pressure on him, he will leave or yield to pressure. When a horse is confined in a small area—a corral or stall, or by a halter or bridle—and feels escape is not an option, he will resist or fight the pressure.

Anytime we have a horse that seems to resist pressure, look for anything that he may think is prohibiting his escape.

If we can open up and give him some more room, then he may find somewhere to relocate and not fight.

For example, when we are trying to move a horse laterally off our leg and he seems to resist the pressure, there was a point he tried to move somewhere, and we blocked him with the reins. He may then think that the only escape route is blocked and start resisting.

We need to understand that when a horse thinks there is no option to escape the pressure, he will go against it. We need to allow the horse to move his feet somewhere, anywhere, then direct the movement in the direction we desire. If we don't have any life in the horse's feet, it is more difficult to direct them. If we first get some movement, then try to direct him, he can learn to associate the direction of movement to the leg pressure. When he responds, give him relief. That will become the escape for him to look for next time.

On the other hand, if a more sensitive horse starts to resist some pressure, and we decrease the pressure or wait and give him more time to look and find an escape, then he doesn't feel like he has to fight. Instead, he feels like he has gotten away from the pressure.

An example of this would be when we ask a horse to respond to a leg. He may respond to some light pressure, but when we increase it, we feel resistance. The horse has the feeling that he cannot out travel the pressure, so it comes back to flight not being an option, and he begins to fight the pressure.

Many times more leg pressure or a harder kick only makes the horse tighten his rib muscles and try to protect himself. When this happens, the horse actually shortens his step instead of increasing it.

Other times, a harder kick will startle the horse and the steps or strides will increase. If the harder kick isn't effective and the length of stride shortens, we may be better off to startle the horse in some other way to increase the stride, like some noise or the end of the mecate on his rump, instead of kicking harder.

Anytime a horse resists pressure, it is not his first choice. Through previous negative experiences he has learned to go against pressure, but that isn't his nature. Only when he perceives a greater pressure will he go against what he thinks is the lesser pressure, and through these experiences, he may "develop" a pattern of going against pressure.

If it was the nature of the horse to go against pressure, a wild mustang would chase you into the trap, instead of you chasing him. But that isn't how it works. He will go to some pretty extreme measures to try and get away from you.

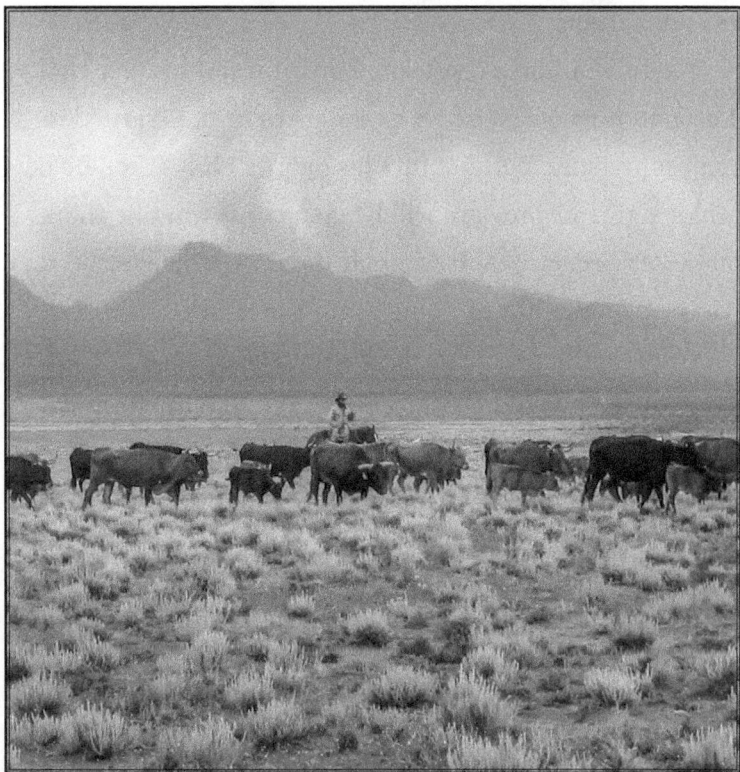

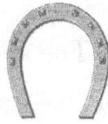

Backing
Up a Hill

If your horse doesn't back up very well, you might find this exercise helpful. If you think your horse backs up well, try backing him up a fairly steep bank and see if he improves or stalls out. If he improves, what you are doing is probably working. If he stalls out, maybe it's because you are doing something that's getting in his way. Here are some things that may help you and your horse.

First off, it would be better if your horse could back a little on flat ground before you ask him to back up a hill, although the procedure is the same to start a horse backing on flat ground as it would be to back up a hill. The slope needs to have good enough footing that he can get ahold of the ground and push with his hind feet without having the ground give way too much. It is OK if he slips some as long

47

as he can move backwards. The angle or grade is not as critical as long as he has reasonable traction; a steeper slope will challenge him more. It would be helpful if the top of the hill or slope has a flat spot so when he is on top, it is a comfortable place for him to rest.

Try riding him forward down the slope, about 6 feet or so, then work him back until he reaches the flat top, then let him relax. The longer he works the longer you should let him rest. If you have any doubt, let him rest longer; too much rest won't hurt this process as much as not enough. A good rule is to let him rest at least as long as he worked.

The first thing to do when preparing to back a horse is to take your weight off the back of the saddle so the horse can raise his loin easier. Just shift your weight to your thighs from your seat bones. I know some people say to lean back to back your horse, but I haven't found one horse that agrees with that theory, and if you put him in a challenging situation like needing to reach back and up, I believe you will find the same thing.

So after your weight is out of the way, start drawing both reins back evenly and slowly. Watch the elevation of the head closely. When the head first starts to raise, hold that amount of pressure, don't increase it, then use one leg, one rein or both on the same side to get the hind-quarters to take one step to the side.

We don't want the front feet to step sideways, only the hind feet. You may need to adjust the position of your rein or leg so you get what is needed and not just a bunch of scrambling around.

When the horse gives you one step sideways with the hindquarters one way, then ask for the hindquarters to step immediately back to the other way, right, left, right, left. At the same time you are asking for the hindquarters to move over, maintain the pressure with the outside rein just enough that he doesn't go forward. If the front end can't go forward and it can't go left or right and the hindquarters stay in motion going left and right, he will eventually look for other options and reach back with the hind foot.

Here is where it is very important that the rider can feel the horse's hind foot reach back because if the horse tries and doesn't get relief for doing the right thing, he will start trying other options that are usually the wrong things and it might take awhile to get back to the right answer. So if you need to have someone watch and call out when the foot sets back, it could be an educational experience for everyone.

Again, whether you start on flat ground, just step the front feet over the slope and leave the hind feet on the flat ground or go down a few steps. Be sure not to measure out too large of a dose that your horse can't find his way out. As he gets more confident with one or two steps, you can ask for three or four.

When you get to the point that the horse steps down four or five steps and backs straight back up the hill with light rein pressure and light alternating leg pressure, see how he feels on flat ground.

When the front feet leave the ground first, it can feel as though you are on a chain being pushed, all the links start piling up in every direction, same as the horse's head, neck, shoulders, ribs and hips. When the hind feet leave the ground first, it feels as though you are on a chain being pulled, all the links are straight. It feels like something is pulling the back of your saddle and the saddle horn is going to come back and hit you in the stomach.

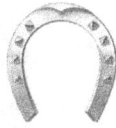

To Spur or Not to Spur?

People often ask about spurs—when or if they should use them. I think it depends on the individual and "when or if" they can control them and "when or if" they are aware of when they are using them.

To me spurs should not be used as the primary signal. First the horse should feel some life or rhythm in our body or legs if we want him to accelerate. If we are asking the horse to move off one leg, we can still put some life in one leg first. If the horse does not respond to the leg or legs, then reinforcement can come with the spur.

Squeezing can be effective. If it is that's fine. The problem that can come from squeezing is that the horse may not realize enough reward. The rider squeezes as the horse's foot leaves the ground and as the foot sets down. Or in another situation when we want to go from point A to point B and we are going to release at point B. But as we depart point A, the horse doesn't get any hint of there being any relief at point B, so he figures why work for point B when there is no sign it is going to be any better than point A. He just learns to tolerate the discomfort. There needs to be some incentive for the horse.

There should be enough respect or even intimidation for the spur that we rarely need to use them. When the horse gets too comfortable with the spur or "desensitized," we can have numerous problems. Besides the obvious that he ignores the request made with the spur, he can get resentful to the point of switching his tail, or even kicking or bucking.

Now, having said that, we must be sure that the horse first understands our request. If we are forcing something on a horse he doesn't understand, we can cause all kinds of problems. He has to understand where we want him to go. It doesn't do any good to hurry if we are headed in the wrong direction. We will just get to the wrong place faster.

The principle of maintaining respect with your spurs is simple: Don't say it if you don't mean it. Like the little kid that learns what "Hot" means, you can warn him to stay away from the hot stove, you can reason with him, explain what will happen, and the more involved you get the more blame and resentment you'll get when he gets in trouble or burned. On the other hand, tell him to stay away from the stove it's "Hot" and if he doesn't, at the peak of his discomfort say "Hot" loud and clear so he clearly understands

"Hot" means pain and discomfort, stay away. If the timing is right and he relates the results to his action, there will be no resentment because he did it to himself. He understands what got him into trouble and what got him out.

As for the spurs, the life in our leg or legs, is the warning "Hot," and the contact with the spur is the burning sensation. We can measure how much we burn the horse; he probably does not need third degree burns on ninety percent of his body. He may not even need a small blister. If a slight red mark is effective and understood, that's all we need. Do what it takes. If you do too much, he may panic. If you don't do enough, you may cause resentment or be ignored totally.

We can start with an increased rhythm in our body, and or fanning or bumping with our calves. If that is not effective, we can then bump him with the side of the stirrup. Sometimes the surprise of a good slap will be effective; a slap on the horse's elbow will have more effect than on his ribs or shoulder. A spank on the rump can also reinforce the meaning of the life in the legs.

The spur should come last and it should be the last thing you say to your horse.

Regardless of what we do to cue the horse, if we ask for something in the same way more than about four times, he will usually start getting desensitized. The first signal should call his attention; the second will measure the response and tell if there needs to be a third and determine if it needs to be less, the same, or more. If it needs to be more, make sure the third time he acknowledges it was more so he doesn't ignore it and get desensitized. If you're not right on, it's better to be on the side of being too strict. You will still have respect. If you are on the side of nagging, you will have resentment.

The horse can be resentful and buck you off or he can get scared and buck you off. Either way the ground can be just as hard. We need to be somewhere in the middle, effective and understood.

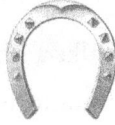

FLAGGING FROM YOUR HORSE

*W*hen I was a boy, the older buckaroos would say "Don't do anything on foot that you can do on horseback." I learned that if you wanted to become a good horseman that was good advice for two reasons. First by trying to do different jobs using your horse, your horse gets handier. Second, the more you do with your horse, the more you can learn from your horse.

With this background when it came to starting horses, it only made sense to me to do all that could be done from a horse. Again, the horse you are riding has a job, so he has an opportunity to become handier. Not only can you be safer and stronger when need be, but you can also become handier.

In recent articles, we talked about the flagging process, the purpose, the philosophy, and now we can talk about the application from another horse. There are two things to remember and maintain using a horse to flag another horse. First, keep your horse's head pointed toward the colt's tail. Second, keep the flag between the colt and your horse as they are in motion. This will be the way to position everything while in motion over ninety percent of the time.

There will be times you may ride straight forward, backup or side pass, but if the flag is effectively working, the colt will be moving away from you. If your horse is traveling toward the colt's tail, the rope will be tipping the colt's nose toward you and the hindquarters away.

Now with those being the primary objectives to positioning, here are some tips that may help. For your horse to travel toward the colt's tail, your rein hand will be pointed toward the colt's tail. When you are working from the right side of your horse, you will be on the right side of the colt. Your reins are in the left hand, and flag in your right hand. When you change sides, change hands. If you don't feel confident and safe with the rope around the saddle horn, hold it in the same hand as your reins. This way as the colt pulls on you, he pulls your rein, turning your horse to catch up. If the colt is pulling too much, raise the flag back over your head away from him to relieve some of the pressure.

As we mentioned earlier, the position of the flag and the angle of the pull on the rope will determine the position of the colt in relation to you. The rope should be adjusted so the colt is at least as far away as your flag can reach. If the colt is responding too much, back off with the flag or give him more rope to give him more distance from you.

If the rope is around the saddle horn, don't tie off solid. Dally and hold the end with your hand or you can tuck a few inches under your thigh or knee with the end of the rope hanging down in front of your leg. If things become unsafe raise your leg and the rope can be released, the dallies will slip and you can be freed from the colt. Safety is always first. You should be familiar and confident with dallying or practice beforehand so you are not attempting to do too many new things at once.

As mentioned in previous articles, the flag is positioned generally between the colt's poll and his loin and between your horse and the colt. This will keep the colt toward the end of the rope and not under your horse's tail. If the colt is bothered by seeing the flag and you allow him to get to your horse's tail, with his head down, he will learn to run under the flag and you will have taught him to hide from it. Don't let this happen. Not only can it be potentially dangerous, it will also make the lesson ineffective.

Working with large animals can be dangerous, especially when they panic and use all their strength. But avoiding trouble can create more trouble. Don't just postpone dealing with the horse's fear; it can confirm his fears and make things worse. Pick your battles, deal with them, but pick the time and place that is favorable and safe for you and your horse. Don't wait and let something happen at an inconvenient and unsafe time.

As discussed in the two previous articles, "Can Your Horse

Survive a Fire Drill" (*Eclectic Horseman* #49) and "Thoughts on Using a Flag" (*Eclectic Horseman* #50), this process will help not only young horses that haven't been handled much but older horses that don't handle a crisis very well. If a horse is braced in the poll and loin, he can learn to soften up. A horse can learn a safe way to respond to frightful situations. He can learn to stop and accept pressure, so he can stand for saddling, picking up his feet, brushing or anything else that may have been bothering him, and causing him to move. Parking your horse is teaching control and is just as important as having control to go right or left, forward or backwards. As a horse learns all this, desensitizing becomes the by-product. A desensitized horse that you cannot control the feet on is, to me, still a dangerous horse.

Obvious things like getting off your horse to open a gate could be made easier after taking some time to learn to do it from your horse. While working cattle in a corral, we can learn to understand cattle and how to work from a horse and make the job better for the cattle by being less stressful, and again you and your horse can become handier.

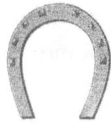

WHAT CAUSES A SORE BACK?

There are a variety of reasons and combinations of things that can make your horse's back sore. Because our horses can't tell us when they are sore or what is making them sore, all we can do is speculate or make an educated guess. Some problems could be more obvious than others, and after seeing some, it may help to educate us to identify a problem in an earlier stage later on with another horse.

Some different things to consider as individuals or in combination would be the load or rider, the saddle and how it fits, the pads or blankets and the horse's condition or shape.

Some people can ride a horse on a long, hot, hard day and maintain a good back, while another rider may take the same horse with the same gear and have problems. In a situation like this with the person being the only difference, we could assume the problem is the way that person rides. For example, some put more weight in the seat or may sit without much rhythm with the horse. I have found this type of rider can experience more problems than someone that rides lighter in the seat with more weight in the stirrups and on their thighs. The more the rider is in time with the horse's rhythm, the less drag or dead weight the horse experiences. This will cause less consistent pressure in a given spot on the horse's back. Some people may have a reason to ride one side heavier than the other. The saddle and horse should be balanced from left to right, and if the rider isn't, this could create a problem.

The amount of weight the horse is carrying can be a factor. When the person starts getting up into the two-fifty-plus pounds they may experience more problems than someone closer to one-fifty. This is where the rhythm plays a big role. Someone weighing one-seventy that rides heavy can cause more damage than a rider that weighs two-forty and rides light.

We also need to consider the horse's condition. If a horse is lean, a saddle may fit fine, but a saddle on the same horse weighing a hundred-fifty pounds heavier with a crease down his back may cause an ill fit, not to mention softer muscles and more heat contributing to the problem.

The shape of the withers in relation to the angle of the bars and the width of the bars on the saddle can be one of the biggest factors. If the horse doesn't fit the saddle we can do only so much with padding, then we may consider the condition of the horse or shape of its back. If the same equipment didn't sore him at one time but then started causing problems later, look at the differences in the horse. Some saddles may work fine and then start soaring a horse. If the bars get warped or broken so the fit changes, this can obviously affect the soundness of their backs.

Thinner high-withered horses generally have trouble on top or on the sides of the withers and they are usually easy to help with cutout pads. Rounder-backed horses can be harder to help when they get fat. The saddle can roll easier so the cinches need to be tighter, which prevents movement and causes more pressure in the same spot.

The horse's back should be reasonably clean. If they are dirty or have longer hair, this can contribute to problems. Clean blankets will also help maintain a good back. Some materials hold dirt more than others, some sweat a horse more than others, some sweat without creating heat and some create heat and may or may not sweat. Vinyl or neoprene sweat without overheating. The old car seats made of Vinyl would sweat you without burning you. Some pads are made with a rubber lining and these can create heat that will irritate a horse's back.

Basically, most of the contributing factors can be narrowed down to two issues: pressure and heat. Pressure in a smaller area can bruise, rub hair and hide off, and decrease blood flow, which can decrease sweating and cause dry spots and callous the hide. Warmer weather is going to contribute to more problems than cooler weather.

Regardless of all the odds that may work against us, there

is one thing that will always help to minimize our problem. If the rider will get off every hour or so depending on the factors previously mentioned and loosen the cinches and raise the saddle up off the horse's back for a few minutes or just unsaddle to allow some circulation to the pressure points and some cool air if their back is hot, this will do as much or more than anything and it doesn't take much time or effort.

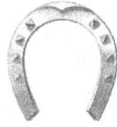

THINK OUTSIDE THE BOXING

*A*fter returning from *The World's Greatest Horse-man* competition, I found it interesting how the contestants handled their cattle in the fence work.

After a lifetime of working cattle and studying how other people handle cattle; how and why they do what they do, I'm sure that it doesn't matter to the cow whether it's at a show or on the ranch. When it is set up a certain way by the rider, it is going to respond accordingly.

Position doesn't always give you a consistent result without analyzing the attitude, temperament and endurance of the cow. The more the cattle are stressed before they come into the arena, the more it will affect them. Reading previous cattle may give you some idea of how yours may work. If they are dehydrated, they will probably be wilder. If they are not relaxed and breathing deep in the back, they will run out of air quicker in the arena and when they don't get enough oxygen to the brain, their decision making isn't as good.

A common mistake made by all levels of competitors in the boxing is to get too close to the cow too soon and show their horse off without considering how it's affecting the cow. This is your free time to shape the cow up for the rest of the run physically and mentally. There is no pattern required and seldom is any credit given in the boxing, but there is a lot of room to gain penalties so this is when it pays for you to be cow smart.

The important thing is to read the flight-zone of the cow, how far away you can be to get the cow to respond. If you can be a third of the way down the arena and the cow is busy responding to you, that may be close enough to start with. Then when you can get control and some rhythm, begin to work in closer. But if you are too close and the cow feels too threatened, it is going to look for a place to escape the trap you have it in and it will try to run past you or it will just run the fence looking for a hole.

The key is to work the cow without causing it to panic. No animal has a thought process while they are panicked; that's the difference between one that's panicked and one that is not. We want them to be thinking so we can read them.

If the cow will come toward the middle of the arena far enough so we can have an opportunity to drive it back to the end and get it to turn back and forth as it is moving forward and away from us, that would be really good.

It doesn't always work to implement mechanical patterns and not read and prepare the cow for what we want it to do the rest of the run. The rest of the run is what will determine your score, and the boxing can have a huge influence.

The remainder of the run would be best if the cow continually turned away from us. If it turns away from us and into the fence, that will give us more time to change sides and stay on the fence to set up the next turn. Then while circling we don't want the cow to be looking toward us, we want it to be moving forward and away. So any opportunity we can shape the cow in the boxing to turn away can help to prepare it for the fence turns and the circling.

When the cow realizes it can turn away and pick us up with the other eye, this can be the first step to a better run. When we are driving the cow, as it prepares to turn away is the time we want to stop and be still until it sees us with the other eye, then turn our horse and shape things up to turn the cow again. If we turn too soon it may keep the cow's attention and it may not want to take its eyes off us.

If the cow feels too much pressure when stopping, it will also look at us and turn into us and there is no place in the rest of the run that will be a positive move. In my opinion credit should be given for the cowboy that can shape the cow to turn away vs. the cow that turns into the horse.

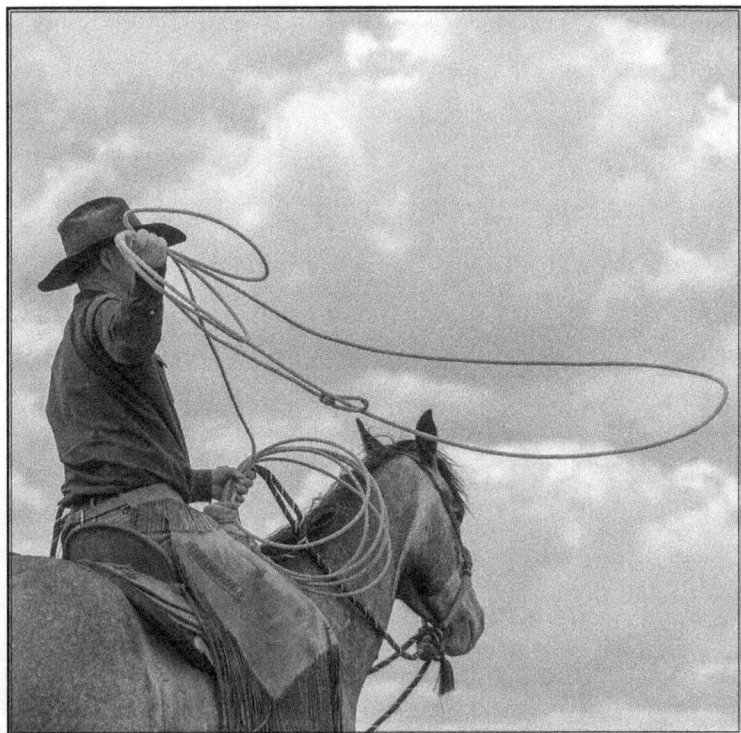

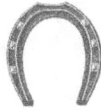

THE MAKING OF A HACKAMORE HORSE

*I*n this modern world of tight schedules we have lost *a lot. One thing being the time it takes to prepare a good hackamore and bridle horse.*

When these horses were made by doing lots of ranch work, without a show schedule deadline, there was no need for short-cuts to get the horses where they needed to be. Like any art, it takes the time it takes; it cannot be rushed.

Two very important things that the hackamore horse needs to be very reliable in is one, to break in the poll in the direction the rein or reins are being drawn, and two, be able to round the loin laterally and vertically with the poll. This does not mean just pulling his nose around to the stirrup. We can bend the head around to the saddle, but the poll may still be tight if the horse is not right mentally.

On the other hand, the horse can tip his poll without bending his neck. When a horse cocks an ear and prepares to cow kick at something, the poll bends and the hindquarter comes in and forward. The loin and poll are bending while the neck and the rest of the horse appear relatively straight, similar to the position a horse may be in when preparing to turn with a cow. This may not be exactly what we are trying to create, but the point is to realize that the horse can flex the important parts of his body without bending other parts. Two things that prevent or make it difficult for the poll and loin to work properly are when the rider has quick or heavy hands. Quick hands can intimidate the horse if the feel and timing are not appropriate. When the horse is intimidated the first thing he is going to do is tighten the poll and possibly engage the flight mode even if for only an instant. This may result in the horse flattening the loin and pushing forward with the hindquarters instead of rounding the loin and pulling with the hindquarters. If the horse needs to collect himself, stop or turn, he will need to round the loin and bend the poll.

The other problem the horse has is the heavy hands of the rider. For a horse to be supple in the poll and light on his feet he needs to have the freedom of his head to balance and shift his weight to move his feet. When the horse has to contend with the extra weight of the rider's heavy hands, it is difficult for the horse to have a relaxed poll. Heavy hands are usually consistent with steady pulling. Steady pulling means the horse has pressure from the rider regardless of whether the foot is leaving the ground or coming toward the ground.

The only time the horse can redirect his weight is when he has contact with the ground. When the foot is committed to coming down it is difficult to change the fall. If I could communicate the direction for you to jump you can comply before you leave the ground, but not after you are airborne. So when the foot is falling we need to have slack in the rein, or relax the pressure, and when the foot we want to direct is on the ground or leaving, we can direct it by making contact with a rein. When the horse understands where we are directing the feet and we understand the timing to draw the reins, it can work beautifully.

This is referred to by many as "pull and slack" or "pull and release," and this allows the horse to stay light to your hands and as a result light on his feet. The poll and the loin work simultaneously the majority of the time. When the horse doesn't feel good to your hands it is probably because he is not positioned correctly in the loin. When you draw the reins the poll should flex and tip the head which shifts the weight and bends the loin, which collects the horse and lightens the front end so he can move easier. It's like a domino effect.

When our timing is right there is no need to pull hard, and when our timing is off we need to pull and release until we find the right timing and not just pull harder. The bigger hammer or pull harder approach doesn't work with a hackamore. It doesn't have the leverage that a bit positioned farther from the poll in softer tissue can. The hands that can maintain a soft hackamore horse will also be able to develop a nice bridle horse the traditional way.

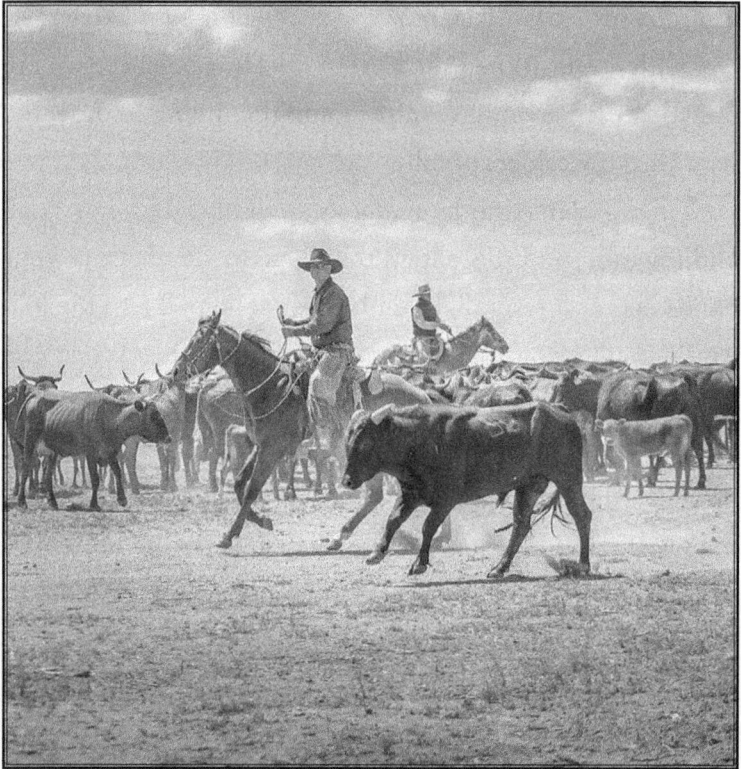

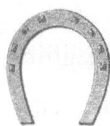

REIN POSITION

*W*hy can one rider have trouble getting a horse to respond and another rider take the same horse and get along great? We may be familiar with the influence of feel and timing, but something that could be quicker for the rider to learn is the effect of the rein or reins in different positions.

We can observe different places we position one or both reins and note the response we get from our horses. Also, note the direction of pull along with the amount and time of pressure applied in relation to the horse's response. It makes no difference whether we wanted the response they gave us. The important thing to note is what action got what reaction.

Experimenting with the following rein positions can potentially give you completely different results: try pulling one rein to your hip, or pulling straight out from the horse's shoulder, in front of the saddle lifting the rein against the wither, or with a short rein lifting and pushing against the jaw. All this is done with one rein, different lengths, different directions and different amounts of pressure, to get totally different responses.

Using one rein to get them to start or stop their feet will get the horse to respond without pulling on our hands as much as they can when we pull on both reins. For example, if we pull both reins evenly to stop and the horse doesn't respond with the feet properly and starts pulling on our hands, we can relax one rein and pull on the other rein enough to put a bend in their neck. Then they won't be pulling as hard as when their neck is straight and this can transmit through the loin to the hindquarter which will step to one side instead of pushing straight ahead, which will help them to slow down.

When backing, if they are heavy, we can take one rein to move the hind feet first, then draw both reins to get the front feet to follow the hind feet back.

Whether it is speed regulation, stop, back, change of direction, or any combination thereof, there is a place that can maximize the message you desire by positioning the rein. Once the horse learns how to interpret our desire and learns how to prepare to do what we are asking, our hands don't need to be in such drastic positions and we can become more uniform with our signals.

Once we understand the effects of one rein, then we can realize the difference when we add the second rein. Again, experimenting with the position and pressure of each rein and all the effects of it; head elevation, speed or change of direction. It is important to identify how the horse places their feet when changing direction. The front quarters can be reaching left while the hindquarters are reaching right, or both front and hind can be reaching the same direction, or one can be neutral, pivoting while the other has all the motion. Also note whether they are in a forward motion or a reverse motion. All of these variations can change because of the position of the rein.

Instead of us trying to force confusing messages on our horses, if we can step back and observe the cause and effect, we learn from that and understand that the horse isn't trying to frustrate us and make trouble for themselves. The horse is always looking for the path of least resistance. Although we may not understand why they do what they do, we can understand what we did to cause them to do it, and use that to get what we want.

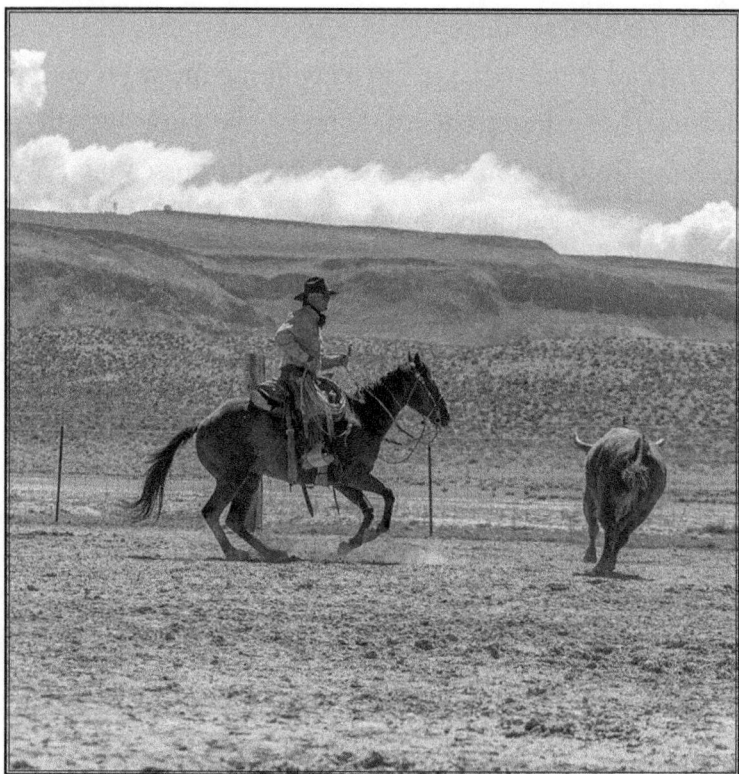

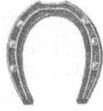

WHAT IT TAKES TO STOP

It is always interesting to me when working with riders to see what they demonstrate when asked to stop their horse.

Some may trot or lope out and perform a nice, soft, straight stop with the horse using his hindquarters, supple from his poll through his hocks, stopping, and then standing quiet and relaxed. That would be my idea of a nice stop, smooth, putting out effort then stand quiet until asked for something else.

What we often see instead is the horse resisting the bridle, stiff in the poll which usually transfers to being stiff through the body down through the legs. Resistance to the bridle can also cause the horse to travel crooked while stopping. If the horse is uncomfortable or worried while trying to stop, he may not stand quiet when asked to stop.

Basically we can have a lot of reasons that our horses don't stop well for us. Pulling harder is often the choice to improve the stop but rarely is that the answer to the problem.

Regardless of what other issues may be in our way of getting a good stop, the one thing that we need is for the horse to stand relaxed and stand quiet when stopped. If the horse stops and then wanders off, or is nervous and doesn't stay in his tracks at the end of the stop he is not thinking stop and will not be preparing and putting the effort into the stop that he could if he were looking forward to some quiet time. Backing a step or two at the end of a stop may help reinforce the horse to pull with the hindquarters, but making it too traumatic can cause resistance and distract the horse's thoughts.

The relief of being stopped can be a major motivator, even softening our hands as the horse shows effort going into the stop can motivate him to think stop. Where more pressure from our hands may discourage and make it difficult for him to stay supple and want to stop. We need to be aware of the energy level in our horse before we school our horse on stopping. When he is in the mood to play and be fresh he will not be thinking stop like he would be if he were a bit tired or needing to air up. If your horse is energetic, use that energy up first then work on stopping and he will appreciate it more. With these things working for you the horse will be mentally ready to stop and he can fill in a lot of other details needed for a good stop.

Some other things that will help are to have the horse moving freely in a straight line when asking to stop. You can be loping a circle or traveling around the arena, but if you just straighten out for just a few strides the horse can stop straight. If the horse is reaching a long full stride, the hind feet will be farther underneath the horse, so when we ask for the stop it will be easier for the horse to use the hindquarters. There are a lot of ways to motivate a horse to stop; some have certain side effects that you may need to deal with later. But if you can make it easy for him to stop with comfortable contact from the bridle, good footing, shoes, and possibly protective leg wear that makes stopping more favorable, then let him stand and relax. The horse will fill in and help us if we make it desirable for him.

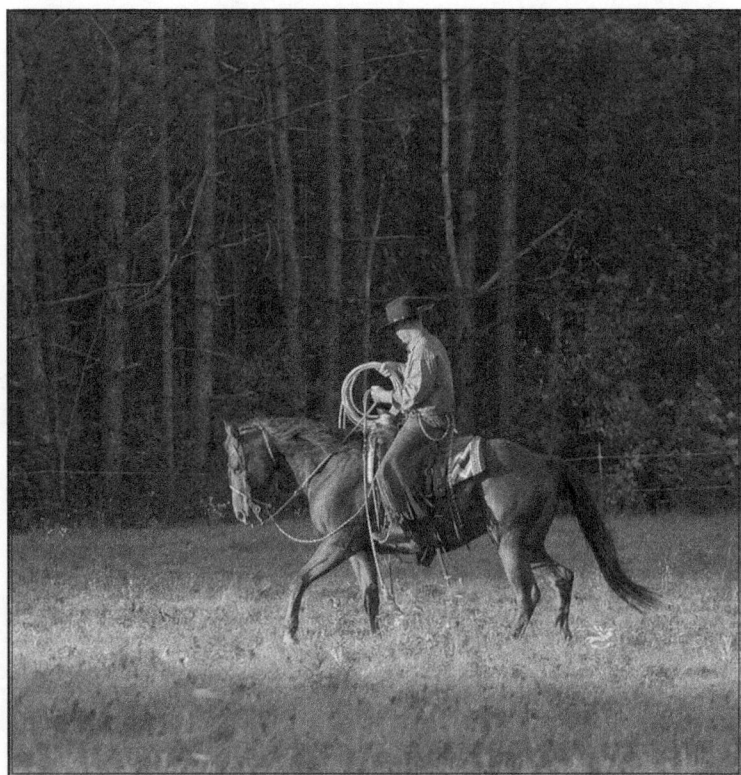

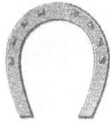

Rating Speed in the Lope

What is important to me, and what I feel is important for a horse, is for him to feel the rhythm of our body and try to be in sync with it. If a horse is not responding to our body rhythm in a slower gait, it can be more obvious in a lope.

You may want to ride slow on a horse that wants to go fast or you may want to ride faster on a horse that wants to go slow. I don't think you should have to be holding a horse to keep him from speeding up or whipping and spurring a horse to keep him from slowing down.

We can start to develop a feel in a walk or a trot by offering the horse a chance to feel our body rhythm. If the horse is traveling slow get your rhythm with the horse then slightly speed your body rhythm up for just two or three strides and if you don't get a slight change, where the horse tries to speed up to be with you, use your legs to kick him or spank him on the butt abruptly, then repeat the process until the horse follows your rhythm.

At first it may not be important that he maintains the speed with you, but what is important is that he makes a change. If he makes a change then you may let him go back to his original speed, then ask again.

If he stays at that speed a few strides and slows down, let him slow down, then repeat the process. This will do two things; it gives you more time to practice making the change which should get him more sensitive to making the change, and it will get him to where he would rather stay with you rather than go through repeating the process of changing.

The same process would apply on a horse that wants to be faster than you want to go. If you are in rhythm with the horse at his pace so he can feel what that feels like, then slow your body rhythm down for a few strides. If he doesn't acknowledge or make a change then take ahold of the reins and get a change, then turn him loose. Once this is working for you slow, then you can start bringing in more speed and work on maintaining the same communication. Again, it is more important for the horse to experience the change than to try to maintain the speed.

Something we want to be careful of is that we don't start the process that I call "boiling the frog." The horse is well aware of the change in our body rhythm; the problem might be that it doesn't have any meaning. All horses like being comfortable. If we make the undesirable uncomfortable by using pressure and we make the desirable comfortable by giving them relief they will be motivated to do the desirable.

The more sensitive we can be to the horse, the more sensitive the horse can be to us. We need to feel the slightest change or try in the horse in order to reward him with comfort when he does what we want and at the same time if he makes a change that we don't want, we need to make it uncomfortable so he will want to change to find a more desirable place to be.

The horse feels our rhythm every stride. He can acknowledge it in one stride, then he can make a change in the second or third stride. But if he goes 4 or 5 strides without the change, that means that you could be getting him desensitized to the feel. This is where it's very important to get a change so the horse understands how and where to get away from the pressure and not just learn to tolerate it.

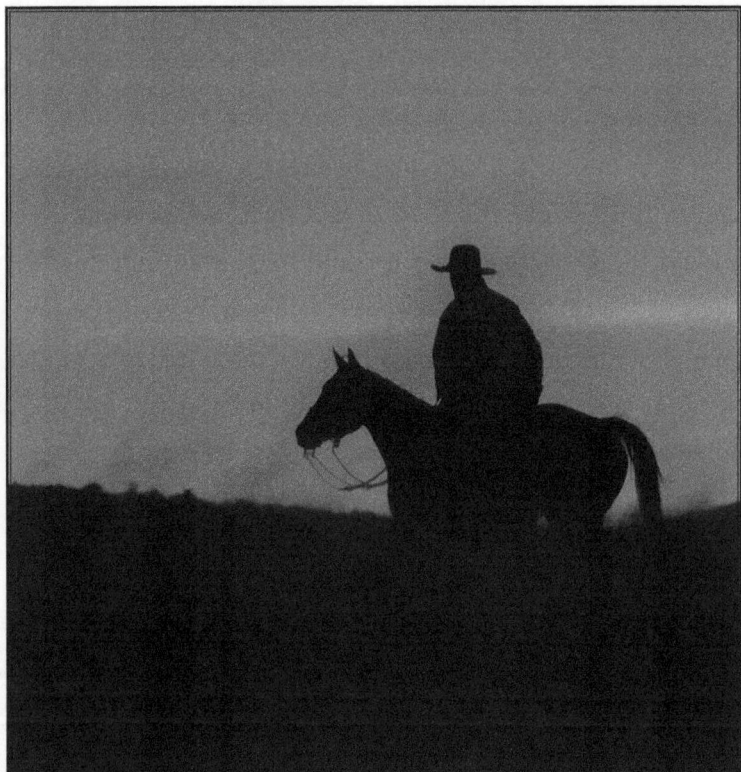

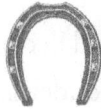

Thumbs Up or Thumbs Down?

We all know that the position of our hands can make a lot of difference on how our horses receive and respond to our reining cues, yet I see very little difference in most riders when it comes to changing the position of their hands if their horse is having trouble. When a person is riding with a rein in each hand, if we notice, their arms may move higher or lower changing the elevation of the hand but the hand itself is in the same position most of the time.

When most people ask for the horse to respond to the reins they may start out with a light pressure, their hands may even be below their hips, their elbows somewhat straight. But if they do not get the response they are looking for they usually pull harder until something changes.

This is like the scenario of one person trying to give instructions to another who speaks a different language. One person talks to the other and because there isn't the expected response, the person gets louder and louder. It doesn't translate any different, the problem isn't that they don't acknowledge you; it's that they don't understand you.

When we can see that our horse is acknowledging our request by trying to do something, then the problem is that they don't understand what we are asking and it's not going to help to ask louder, only cause confusion, anxiety or fear. If we continue to ride this way, eventually most horses will become calloused.

If our horse is acknowledging us and if they don't respond correctly in a reasonable amount of time, we need to change our message in some way so that it makes sense to them. This doesn't just mean bring our hands to our hips so we have more leverage.

The direction our thumbs are pointing, especially when it comes to lateral movement, but also when we are stopping, backing or steering them straight forward, can make a huge difference.

For example, when our thumbs are pointed out, our elbows are in next to our side and we are using our biceps. This means we are more likely to lock our arms and be very firm with our hands. When the horse feels this they will usually react by pulling against us because their only choices are to either put their chin on their chest where they can't go any farther or pull an equal amount of pressure in order to maintain their head position and their balance.

When the thumbs are pointed up we can offer a slightly different feel, a little softer, but we are still using our biceps mostly so the affect is going to be similar to our thumbs pointed out. Our elbows are still next to our side where it is easy for us to lock up and we will likely resort to using strength rather than finesse, causing the horse to react by going against the pressure.

When our thumbs are pointed in with our palms down, we are using more triceps and less bicep, making it less likely to lock our arms. This, as a result, makes our hands softer which is going to help maintain softness in our horses.

If we point our thumbs down and straighten our arms on a less experienced horse or one that has trouble getting enough forward motion, it can be very helpful. This means that we are either lifting our arm and or pushing it out; in either case we will not be using any bicep and we cannot put as much pressure on the reins. We can't teach the horse to resist as much pressure if we are not putting the pressure there for him to experience. Instead, we are offering a softer feel and giving the horse more time to move into our hands because our hands are in a leading position instead of a blocking position.

Whether you are using one rein at a time or both to point the horses' nose, try riding with your thumbs pointed in and see if it doesn't soften your horses. If you are having trouble getting forward motion, point your thumbs down and your palm out to the side and see if your horse will get to moving forward better for you.

There still may be times you need to point your thumbs up or out, but save that for when all else fails instead of your first response.

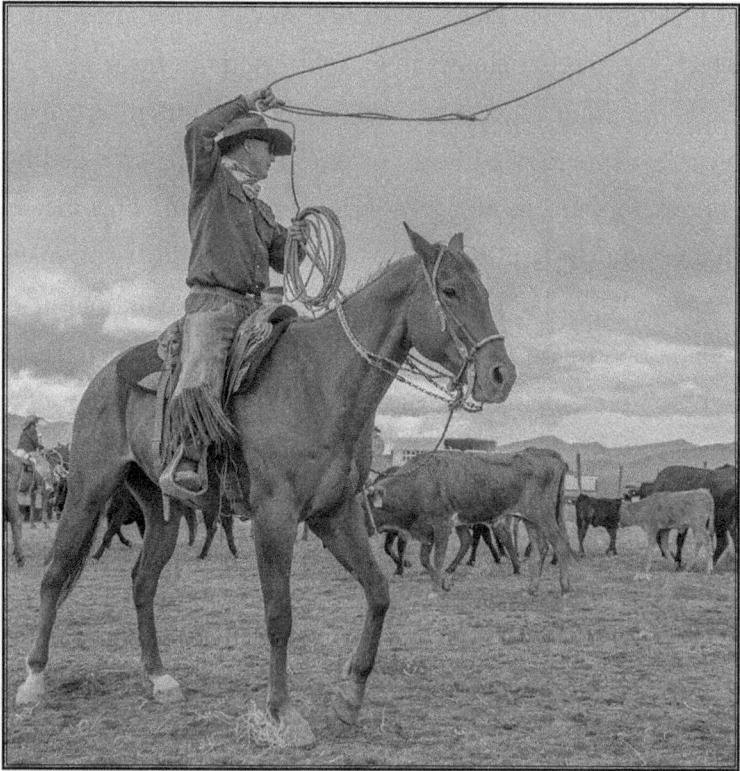

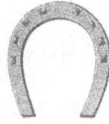

Turn Tail To a Cow

G rowing up and working around horsemen all my life I have heard as much as anyone to never turn tail to a cow. It was interesting when I was in Australia to hear the stockmen there ruled the same as the stockmen in America on this subject. "If a horse is going to learn to watch a cow he can't do it with his tail etc." Knowing full well a lot of old-timers (including my grandfather and great-grandfather) would roll over in their graves, and the living would burn this writing I am going to say there are exceptions to this rule and would advise being open-minded enough to at least consider.

One scenario would be on a real green horse in working conditions (in other words not good training conditions, brush, obstacles, tough cattle, etc.) When the horse may be rating the cow holding it out of the herd, this should be somewhat a comfortable experience encouraging the horse to be in that position. Then the cow ducks under the horse's tail and goes back to the herd. Now the cow prepared, made the call, and executed the move, which may have been a 90 degree change of direction. Now the horse can try to stop, which if he is green would take some distances, then turn 270 degrees, then have to hustle to make up the distance and try to rate back when and if you catch the cow before it gets back to the herd. If it does beat you to the herd instead of all that maneuvering, turn away or what we call, turn tail. If the cow was on your left side and ducked behind your horse, it would now be somewhere behind and to the right. If you turn right 90 degrees without stopping you would be somewhat paralleling the cow's line of travel and likely be consistent with its speed. You are in a position to push the cow to the right in a quarter circle and end up on your original line of travel perpendicular with the herd.

If we are on a green horse that doesn't stop or turn good enough, we can school them with some better-quality reining by turning tail, and when the horse gets handy enough or the cow gets slowed down enough, then we can turn into the cow, "like we are supposed to." This way the young horse is experiencing more time comfortable and in position with the cow and less time confused and out of position. Often I see the horse hurried to stop and turn with his head in the air thinking about keeping his feet under him and the last thing he is thinking about is "watching a cow."

Also, if it means anything, the cow experiences less relief time from the horse. The more relief the cow gets, the harder it is going to try to get away the next time the situation shapes up. By turning tail, depending on how quick you get back into position to pressure it to the right, the cow can have little if any time to experience relief.

Another scenario would be when the cow is on a line of travel and very determined to maintain it and may not have much yield of speed either. Maybe you are in a valley, a canyon, or just a trail of some kind that the cow doesn't want to give up. This would apply the same as the previous scenario except instead of saving a 270 degree turn to make a 90 degree turn, you may be saving closer to a 360 degree turn and maintaining the same line of travel, and speed. Many times in this situation if you can't turn the cow around, the next best thing would be to swing the cow as far to the right as possible waiting for it to slow down. Then if it does duck behind, swing it to the left as much as possible waiting for it to slow down. Eventually if you maintain a certain amount of pressure and keep offering it a place to stop, the cow can learn to yield to your pressure by stopping. If you can't stop a cow, you really don't have control of her.

Chances are the cow is out of air by now, but not as determined to go by you obviously if it stopped. It is either thinking about finding a better way to deal with you, or it is so tired it can't move. In either case time would be on your side. The longer you wait for her to move, the better chance it will make a move to yield from you. The cow is going to need time to process its thoughts of yielding to the pressure that stopped it, which could relate to yielding to some pressure to turn it a different direction, or if the cow gives out it will obviously need time to air up and restore enough energy to go again. Either way the more you hurry, the longer it may take.

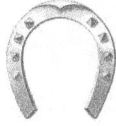

FOOTFALL OF A TURNAROUND

With the growing interest in Ranch Horse competitions, Cow Horse events, and people just wanting to advance their horsemanship to a higher level, one maneuver that seems to give people difficulties is the turnaround.

To some people a turnaround is merely a turn on the haunches, but if we are going to expect precision and speed, it needs to be more specific than that. If we know where the feet are and if they are where and how they need to be to get them arranged the way we need them, it can be very simple, but if not it can be frustrating, right?

In order for the horse to turn in place he needs to maintain a specific pivot foot to prevent them from drifting. He can go forward around an inside pivot point foot, or he can go backward around an outside pivot foot, or he can switch back and forth. In any case, if he is pulling with the hind-quarters against the front end he creates centrifugal force and that creates speed.

This may seem very detailed to a person, but if we understand a horse's movement, positive or negative, and the cause and effect we have on him, then we can affect him in a positive way and not cause any negative... hopefully. We can make the wrong movement uncomfortable and the right movement comfortable for our horse, but only when we understand what's right or wrong. The horse needs to be able to stay balanced and use his strength to execute speed. We need to be very clear so he can move correctly for what we want and not get him confused as to what we want him to do. If we consider how the horse naturally moves it is easier to allow him to do a maneuver to the best of his ability.

Let's look at the difference in the foot placement as a horse walks forward, then we will look at the foot placement as a horse backs up. If you need to familiarize yourself, spend some time watching a horse as he is walking to get a better idea of the sequence of his footfall. Then as you read the following, try to get a picture in your mind of the footfall as the horse is turning in a forward motion.

At a walk, the left hind foot comes forward and down as the left front foot is leaving the ground more or less depending on how fast he walks and how far he reaches with the hind foot. At this point if we draw the left rein as the left front foot leaves the ground in a way that brings the foot to the left, and at this same time with the same rein we stop the forward motion and hold the left hind foot in place, this means in a left turn the left hind foot is up underneath the horse and stays there.

As the left front is coming down, relax the pressure of the rein and just give him a feel to follow. As the left front is coming down the right hind is off the ground coming forward and around the left hind, then as the right hind comes down the right front leaves the ground and comes forward and around in front of the left front foot. As the right hind foot is in motion just maintain a soft rein. Too much pressure at this point will cause a right hind foot to step out. Wait until the left feet are in motion and then repeat the complete process.

If we hold the rein too long and don't allow the other three feet to come forward the left hind foot may step back. This not only can cause the hind legs to have trouble but it can also cause trouble with the front foot placement.

Now for the foot placement as a horse is backing up. When a horse backs up, the left front is off the ground more or less as the right hind is off the ground. A horse backs in diagonals. Another thing to note is the front leg can only reach sideways a minimal distance, the shoulder blade can extend forward and can go back, but it does not come directly sideways very far. This means the horse can't bring the front foot to the side very far. To reach very far he will be moving forward or backing.

If we try to bring the left front leg back and out to the left this puts a horse in a backing footfall, which means as the left foot is coming back and out to the left it's likely for the right hind to reach back and out to the right. If this happens we are basically disengaging the hindquarters and taking the power away from him. In order to utilize centrifugal force to get speed in the turn, a hind foot needs to be pulling against the front end. He cannot do this if he is disengaged. Horses are limited to how fast they can reach to the left with the front end and to the right with the hind end.

This explains the difference in a forward and a backing tur. Next time we will discuss where each type of turnaround would be most applicable. There are reasons for both, and especially in cow work a horse needs to be able to do both.

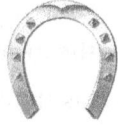

Pivot Foot

Just asking a horse to turn on the hindquarters, or haunches, can leave a lot of unanswered questions and confusion for the horse. If we can first understand the horse's foot position as they are turning around on their hindquarters, and realize what would be the most useful way for him to place his feet for what we need, then we can help him to position his feet for a better turn.

A horse can pivot on one hind foot and step the other hind foot forward, or back, or sideways. He can step forward with the outside foot and back with the inside foot, or he can hop in the air with both to reset them both as he turns. And what the hind feet do can affect and limit what the front feet can do.

Starting with the natural movement of the horse, let's study the footfall as a horse walks forward and as they back up. As discussed in an earlier article (*Eclectic Horseman* #80) the front left foot is leaving the ground as the hind left foot is setting down, more or less, as they walk forward. The front foot can come left as the hind foot sets forward giving us an inside pivot foot.

When they are backing the feet leave the ground in diagonals. The left front would leave with the right hind. This means as they step back we need to be aware that bringing the left front foot to the left can cause the right hind foot to step to the right because of the foot being unloaded and needing to balance his weight shift. If we ask the front end to come left as the right front leaves the ground, the left hind would be unloaded and can step back. Depending on how far he steps back the horse may not be able to cross over in front of the left front as the right front is in the air. He may step short to avoid hitting the left front, or he can reach behind the left front with the right front. This takes a lot of practice for the horse to learn where to place his feet when speed is added to the equation because he relates speed to forward motion.

In order for a horse to turn with speed he needs to understand to step with a forward motion with his front feet, and backing motion with the hind feet. It can be a problem accomplishing this with speed and precision for a spin. Typically, the horse tries different alternatives; he may hop or lope around with both front feet off the ground at the same time, he may bump or step on himself and if he doesn't learn to reach back well, he drags his feet.

It's not that difficult for a horse to back with the front and hind. While turning as the hind steps back and over to the right, it gives the front room to come back and over to the left, all while moving away from the cow. And because this type of turn helps to slow the cow it will give the horse a chance to turn slower. For position on a cow this is a very practical turn. The horse can relate it to moving with and away from the cow and not need to depend on the rider completely to be motivated to position themselves.

If we look closely the top cutting horses in competition, the hind steps outside their line of travel to make room for the front to come back and through. Both hinds are loaded to stop, then as they complete the turn the inside hind takes more load to hold the pivot as the outside comes around and they both launch them forward. The outside is setting out to position and the inside is propelling speed and forward motion.

A horse should be able to turn either direction on either hind foot to have a balance in his ability to execute the appropriate turn for the occasion. Horse racing history has long established the fact that horses have the ability to move fastest with forward motion. But when we are turning with a cow and we are moving toward her, she is more likely to speed up than if we are moving away.

It is my observation, the outside pivot foot is for position, the inside pivot foot is for speed. They both have their place.

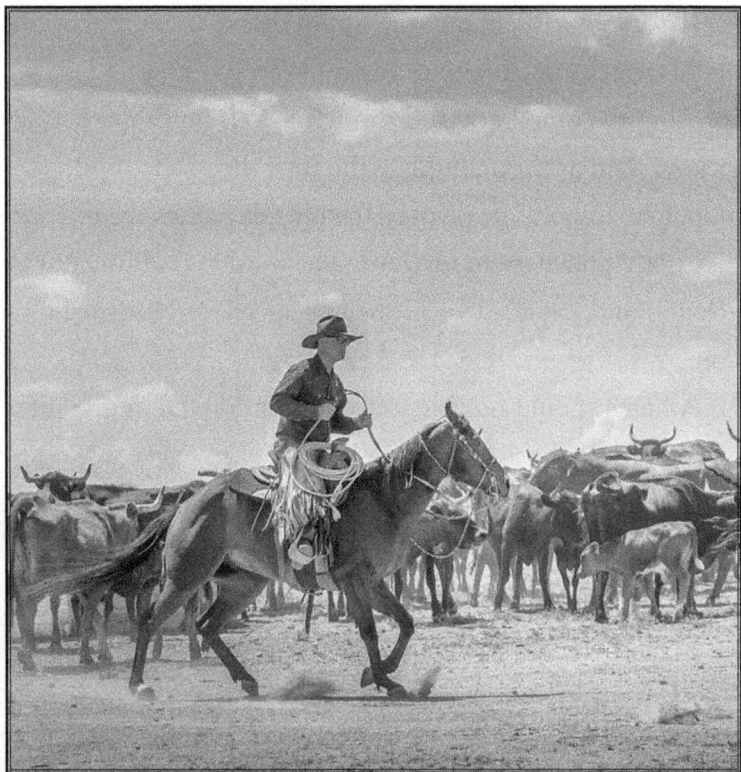

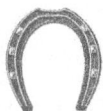

HAND POSITIONS–
IN AND OUT OF THE BOX

*E*verybody learned when they were starting out to keep your hands down low, pull back toward your hip, and keep your elbows in, right? Keep your hands inside a box some say. And that is exactly right part of the time. That's what I want in a bridle horse, both reins in one hand and not moving but only inches around the saddle horn, in the END.

But that can be exactly wrong a lot of the time also especially if we are working with horses that are unfamiliar with how, or are unwilling, to operate with that kind of handling. So that's not where we START.

If we have a younger inexperienced horse, or the older horse that has learned to get heavy, quite often from that kind of handling, we don't need to stay in the box. When things are right, and the horse understands our hands they can be close to the withers, but too often when that doesn't work the next solution is to pull harder, instead of changing the position of the hands, or getting out of the box.

When the horse gets out of control most people understand to use one rein to get the horse stopped, or back in control. But let's define out of control. When you have to pull hard enough that you need to close your fingers to grip the reins, that's my definition of losing control.

Once we brace our biceps and the horse braces his neck, it's a matter of time before that perpetuates into him pulling more than we can. To me that's out of control. "The only way a horse learns to pull on us, is for us to pull on him and teach him how strong he really is. The only strength a horse learns to use against us, is what we teach him through resistance."

A problem when we are pulling one rein is if we don't release the outside rein and we are still pulling back to our hip with the inside, we may be limited in getting the benefit of controlling the horse. This is why we only see limited success with this method quite often.

What a lot of people have trouble with is completely letting go of the outside rein, and raising the inside rein farther up the horse's neck, and coming out away from the neck so it's somewhat perpendicular to the jaw of the horse.

This seems awkward because we're using our triceps more than our biceps. We are not as strong but the horse is not as strong opposing us at this angle either. It goes against everything previous instruction has taught us, and our instincts. People may feel they need to pull steady till they get stopped, and if it's taking too long, "pull harder."

If we can find a position that tips the nose out and slightly up, then wait on the feet, releasing the pressure when the horse rebalances, it will make sense and be comfortable to the horse. The position of the hand through the rein affects the position of the nose; the position of the nose through the neck positions the body; the position of the body through the legs positions the feet. In short, "We can't get the feet in position if the hands are out of position."

We just need to convince ourselves to reach forward toward the ear, with a short rein, push the rein out and up with the palm out, put pressure on the rein but then soften it in time with the horse. "Bad timing is better than no timing"; at least the horse may get in time with us. But they can't get in time with steady pressure and that makes them heavy. They can learn to find the release by getting drug through a maneuver, but rewarding each step is much more effective.

Don't be afraid to explore for a hand position that your horse might be lighter and more responsive to.

Your instructor might tell you what's wrong, but the horse will tell you what's right.

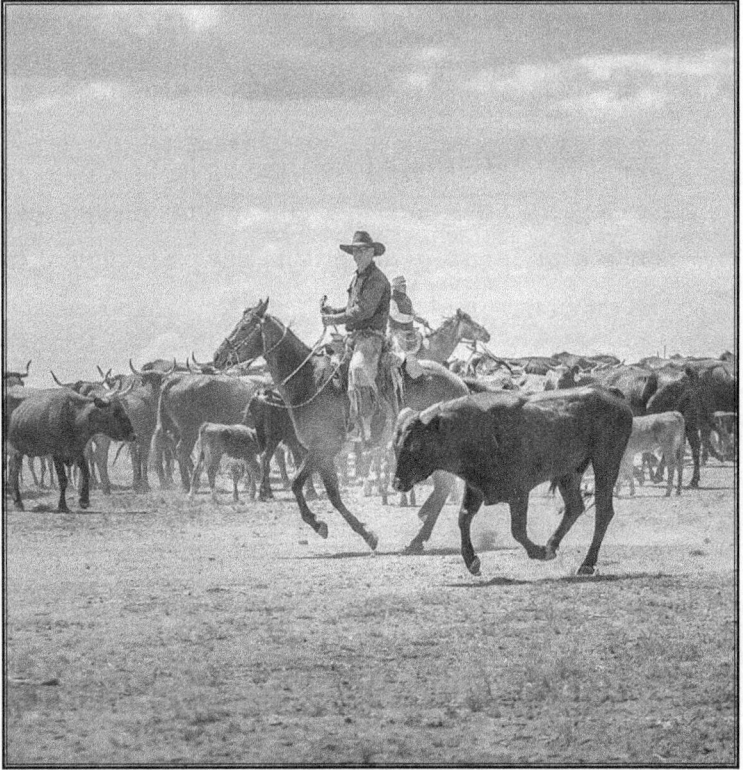

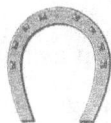

A THIRD,
A THIRD, A THIRD

Sometimes I'm asked where I put my weight in the saddle in relation to my legs, my seat, and my thighs. There's not many things I do "just because" or, "that's what I've been told." Even if it is correct I want to know what makes it correct so I understand. So here's what I do and why I do it; there are other ways of doing it and reasons for doing it other ways.

The lighter we are in the seat, the easier it is for a horse to move. The heavier we are in the seat, the more effort it takes for the horse to move. So if we want to make it easier for the horse we can increase the weight in our stirrups and thighs and decrease the weight from our seat. This may take some conditioning for some riders that just want to sit in the saddle like they are sitting on a chair. It may take some muscle toning so their legs don't get tired.

If we want to discourage the movement in a horse we can decrease the weight in the stirrups and thighs and increase the weight in our seat. Most riders that ride heavy in the seat will have slower moving horses. So if we want a horse to travel slower we can sit heavier.

This is like the toddler when they want picked up. They rise up and get taller and when we get ahold of them, they are ready to get with us and are easier to pick up. But when they don't want picked up they slouch down and get real limber and feel considerably heavier and harder to pick up. I think it's the same way for a horse if we try to get with them or if we are making it hard for them to get with us.

We can use this as a cue to help stop our horses. If we have a lot of rhythm with them when we want them to be traveling, then we get heavy in our seat even before picking our reins up, they notice that.

It's important for horses to be in the rhythm, it's part of their survival. When they run to the herd to avoid a perceived predator, they get in sync with the other animals. If they didn't they would be crashing into each other and the predator could catch them easier. They also try real hard to get in rhythm with us. We may have to work at this, but they come by it naturally, without even thinking about it.

So, if we can ride with about a third of our weight in the seat, about a third on the thighs, and about a third in our stirrups, I believe this gives them a good feeling. Then if be want to increase the horse's rhythm, lighten our seat and possibly our thighs and increase the weight in our stirrups. This brings our center of gravity forward and makes it easier for the horse to take us.

There's other reasons why a horse may be faster or slower than a person likes; but if we decrease the weight in our stirrups and increase the weight in our seat it makes it harder for the horse to have a good rhythm with us. If we roll back against our tail bone, bring our pelvis up and forward and take our shoulders back, raise our knees until we hardly have any weight in the stirrups, the horse will generally slow down.

Like the old saying goes, "ride a fast horse slow, and a slow horse fast." They will even out.

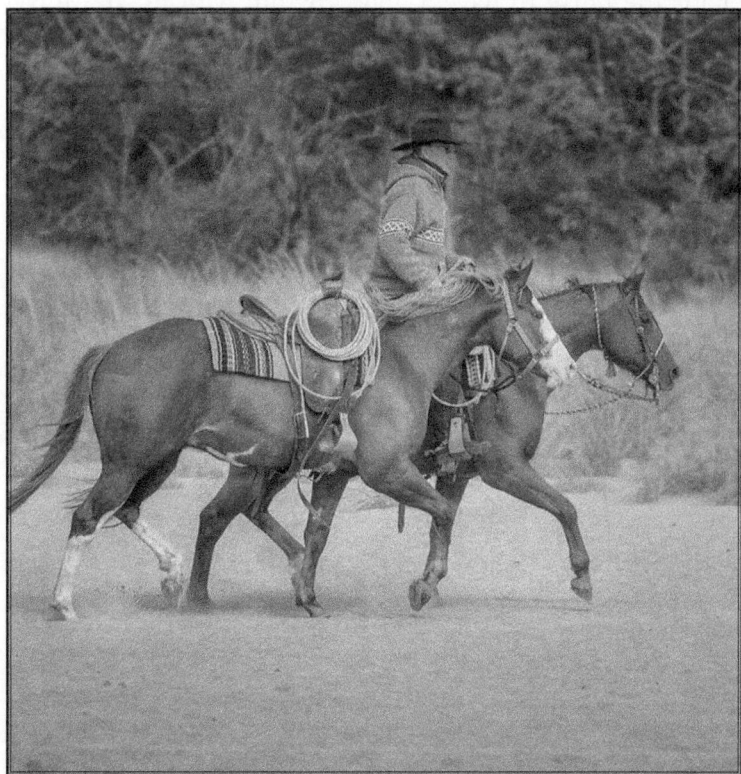

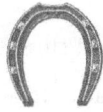

Inside Rein - Outside Leg

That's not a new concept. But what does that mean?

I guess it can mean different things to different people because I see many different applications of it. Quite often I see horses that overbend in the neck; in other words, if the outside rein is not there to stop the horse from overbending the horse's ribs go out against the outside leg.

There is a balance to everything. We can have too much of a good thing and create a bad thing. We need the bend in our horses to direct them in a balanced way, but we can get them too soft and supple to the inside rein to the point that we have to have an outside rein to stop them from over bending.

If we have the feel to acknowledge the horse preparing, and wait so the horse can perform for us without our doing too much, we can prevent creating problems. We only need to start the horse in the right direction and then release. This is where timing is important. If we have the timing we can acknowledge each step and direct each step as necessary. We draw the inside rein and with our outside leg we put life in the feet and release when they respond, then repeat this with the next step. Steady pressure makes horses dull and heavy, pressure and relief in the right proportions with the feet is what keeps a horse light and responsive.

What I see is the inside rein might be the primary rein, but when it causes the hindquarters to move out the opposite direction, the outside rein becomes just as effective to prevent overbending the horse.

If we pull the inside rein back or out too much we can easily create too much bend. Also when this happens the horse usually ends up ignoring the outside leg to whatever extent while trying to stay balanced by stepping the hindquarters out.

If we position the outside rein across the neck to push the shoulder we can create a counterbend, restrict forward motion, and just confuse the horse and make them resistant. Then we can get too much pressure on both reins, the outside leg, and possibly the inside leg when forward motion becomes a problem caused from the pressure of both reins, and then we can have horses that are heavy and dull from all the rein and leg pressure.

When we have too much effect from the outside leg on the more responsive horse, it can create bend in the poll to the outside tipping their nose out, putting them in a counterbend, and they can be off balance. This can make the horse stiff in the jaw and neck and can result in a heavy and dull horse.

But then quite often the solution for the heavy or dull horse to our reins is to flex the horse to get the soft feel again. Then the horse is refreshed on being suppled and giving to the inside rein again, and the cycle continues.

Think of the inside rein to only direct the horse and the outside leg to drive the horse. This means only the inside rein positions the horse's head and neck. The position of the rein can be more important than the amount of pressure. If the rein is out and or back too much, it can cause too much bend. If the rein is forward and up slightly, the neck and shoulders can stay straighter and lighter to the inside hand.

If we learn to measure out just the right pressure in just the right position, the outside rein will not be needed.

Here's a very simple test of our feel, timing, and balance, in my opinion. Simply put your outside hand on the horse's neck with a loose rein while you raise the inside rein up close to the horse's neck without doing enough to cause too much bend, and wait. Then lightly put some outside leg on your horse to create forward motion toward your inside rein.

This simple request can answer several things with your horse and how you are communicating with them. If they haven't been overflexed, their front feet should go toward their nose and the hind feet toward their front. With the inside rein and outside leg, only!

You can grade your own paper.

Can you position the head where you only see the inside eyelashes without using the outside rein to stop the bend?

Can you start forward motion with your outside leg without the shoulder falling outside or inside of the directions of the nose? To me when we can find just the right proportion of influence with the inside rein and the outside leg, nothing else is needed.

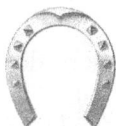

WHAT'S THE FIRST STEP?

In previous articles we have talked about turn arounds and the exercise of pivoting on each of the four feet. Like a lot of things we ask our horses to do whether it is turning around, or any other foot placement, it is important to realize what takes place before what we are asking for takes place.

Horses are quick to get in the habit of responding a certain way when we ask them to do things. For example, when we put a leg on our horse's side the majority of the time it is for forward movement. As a result; if we lay one leg for lateral movement we are likely to cause the horse to go forward into the bridle even when the horse may have already acknowledged our hands ready to block forward movement. If we want our horses to be handy and have a clear understanding of the cues we use to direct them we need to work on ourselves to be clear and precise when asking for something.

If we want to step the front end over the first step or two should be the front end not the hind feet and the front end should step over not forward. This is where we can be more clear and precise. If we are not getting what we ask for when we ask for it, we may need to train ourselves to be more aware of what is preparing to happen before it happens. When we allow the horse to take some steps forward then use our hands more to stop the forward motion, then use more rein to try to move the front end over and the hind end falls out, then the front end steps over what are we teaching our horse? They are quick to pick up a pattern from misunderstanding what it is we really were asking for.

We need to allow all these wrong answers and make it clear what the correct answer is. We need to realize that the horse is doing what he is doing because that is how he understands our cues. The more we allow the miscommunication, the more difficult and frustrating it can be for both horse and rider to straighten out as time goes on.

When we ask for the front end to step over, feel if the saddle horn is starting to shift forward or over. Before the horse moves their feet forward, the saddle horn is going to move forward, you don't need to know where the feet are or what they are doing necessarily to realize what direction the saddle horn is moving.

If the first movement is forward don't press harder with your leg, its not that the horse didn't hear you, it didn't understand what you said. Start over and this time shift the saddle horn backward an inch or two then ask them to move the front end over. This will allow the horse to understand moving the front end doesn't necessarily need to associate with moving forward.

You can practice moving the hindquarters the same way. We should learn to communicate exactly which quarter to move which direction with out some extra steps shifting directions we don't want or need.

Again, we need to realize what the horse is doing is their interpretation of our message. If it's wrong we need to accept the responsibility and try a different presentation to get a clearer message.

www.ingramcontent.com/pod-product-compliance
Lightning Source LLC
Chambersburg PA
CBHW031521270326
41930CB00006B/461